BECOMING
BULLETPROOF

HOW TO BECOME RESILIENT TO STRESS IN AN ERA OF ANXIETY

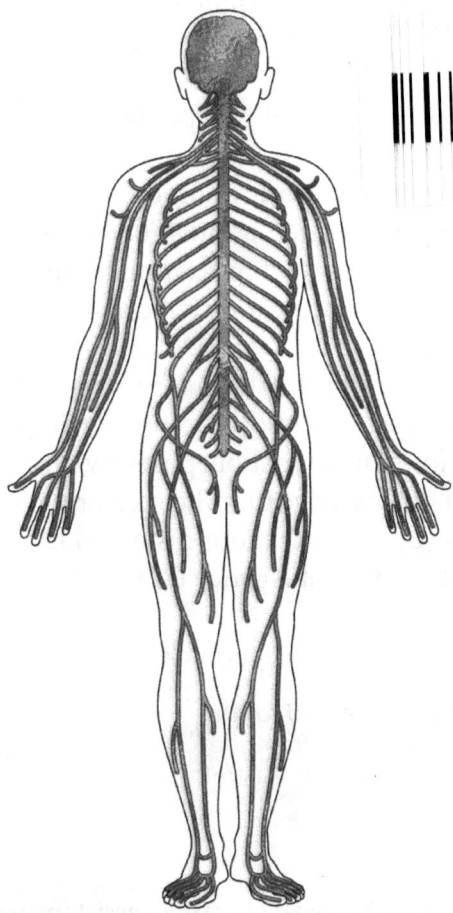

I0095812

WILL WARREN-DAVEY

Becoming Bulletproof: How to Become Resilient to Stress in an Era of Anxiety

ISBN: 978-1-923163-04-1 (Paperback)

NATIONAL LIBRARY OF AUSTRALIA A catalogue record for this book is available from the National Library of Australia

Self-Published by Will Warren-Davey with assistance by Clark & Mackay

Proudly printed in Australia by Clark & Mackay

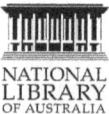

NOTES FROM THE AUTHOR

THIS BOOK HAS been a real passion project, albeit one also fuelled by a feeling of moral obligation.

This moral obligation comes from being an active observer and coming to the conclusion that stress is the default setting of modern society.

For nearly 10 years, I have travelled the countryside, giving seminars, workshops, talks, and recommendations to people to help give a psalm for the modern condition – stress.

I have first-hand witnessed for years the health of literally hundreds of people decline from the crushing burden of chronic stress. This singular mission is why I have authored this book.

The intention of my entire career has been to help improve health on as large a scale as humanly possible. To create a positive impact on the health of the population at large.

To give a toolkit to those who struggle day in and day out with declining health from the silent killer that's literally screaming at deaf ears – stress!

My only hope is that this book serves as a resource to help improve health and the quality of life for you reading along at home.

For the everyday battlers out there trying to keep up with the crazy pace of modern life, this book is a bible built specifically for you!

I hope by making this text available, we can all start to see the biological writing on the wall and take action today to help make you bulletproof to the immense pressures of modern living!

DEFINING BULLETPROOF

As the title of the book may have given away, the goal of this book is to show you how stress impacts every aspect of your body, both positively and negatively.

But this is only half of the equation!

The true mission of the book is to inform you of the dangers of chronic stress and educate you on its impact, and then to give you the tools to become resilient to that stress and thrive and not just survive!

For the purpose of this book, being 'bulletproof' therefore refers to becoming physiologically resilient to the negative effects of stress on the body.

Resilience in all areas is the true goal of biology!

Resilience is how your immune system can fend off foreign invaders, viruses, pathogens, and infections.

Resilience is how your body can bounce back from physical stressors placed upon it, whether that is from exercise or your physical job.

Resilience within your primary sex hormones like testosterone and estrogen ensures that you remain hormonally optimised, even in the face of biological adversity.

Mental resilience can enable you to maintain motivation and drive and enjoy peace, joy, fulfilment, and ambition throughout the challenges of modern living.

Last, but definitely not least, comes forging resilience in your metabolism as it is assaulted by the contemporary default – chronic stress.

PART 1

A SYNOPSIS OF THE STRESS OF THE MODERN CONDITION

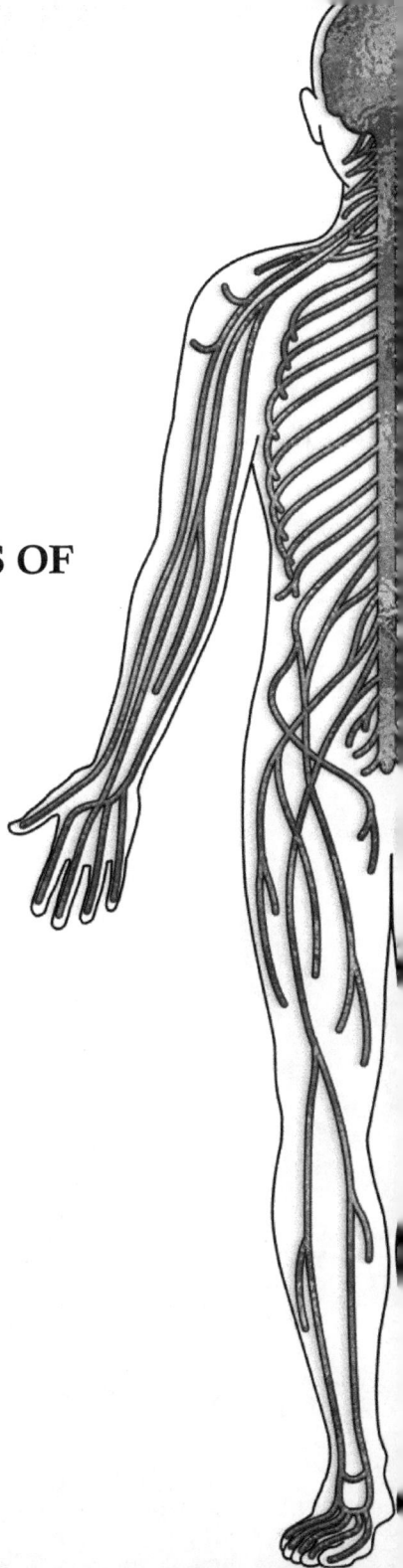

CHAPTER 1

AN OVERVIEW OF STRESS PHYSIOLOGY

IT IS FASCINATING how the body can adapt to nearly anything!

The human body is an incredible machine capable of enduring immeasurable extremes, both chronically and acutely, in the name of its ultimate priority-survival!

The purpose of this book is to give you an understanding of and appreciation for the wondrous thing that is the human body!

And in so doing, to give you a more thorough understanding of how stress works in your body so we can in turn help you achieve the mission of this book making you bulletproof to stress!

SO HOW DOES YOUR BODY RESPOND TO STRESS?

To make you bulletproof to stress, we must be able to clearly define what stress is and identify the way our stress hormones, such as adrenaline and cortisol, play out in the body in the face of a stressful time.

Whilst in this book, we are focusing in many instances on the negatives of cortisol and other associated stress hormones, but before we dive in, I just want to make it clear that Cortisol is a necessary and powerful hormone that regulates a host of areas including:

- Energy Production
- Metabolism and blood sugar regulation
- Blood Pressure
- Heart Rate
- Immune Function
- Reproductive Hormones

Without it, we would literally die.

It is a master regulator of almost every system in the body and when it's working as it should, it's our best friend in so many ways!

It is only when it becomes chronically elevated above normal levels and stays elevated that we start to see the wheels fall off the stress-fuelled apple cart.

NORMAL CORTISOL RHYTHM AND FUNCTION-CIRCADIAN FUNCTION

This diagram from the *Psychology in Action* journal is a great illustration of how cortisol is meant to work in a perfect world.

This curve is what we refer to as a diurnal curve, characterised by an increase in the morning and a decrease in the latter half of the day.

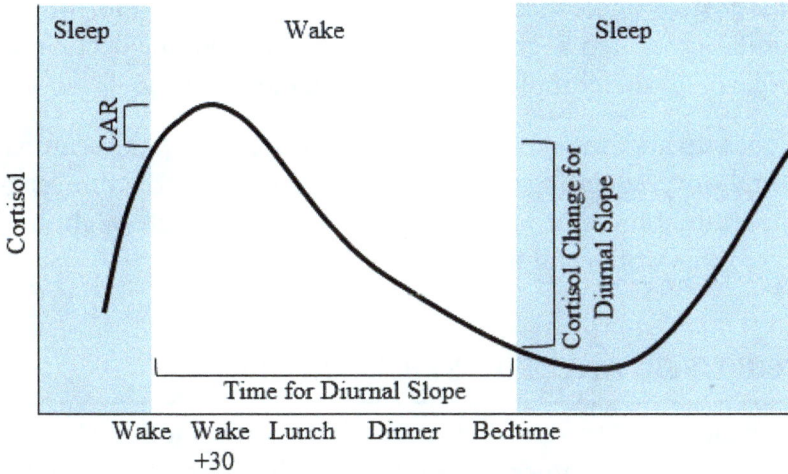

Figure 1 – An illustration of a healthy cortisol rhythm in its diurnal patterns. Cortisol is meant to spike in the first half of the day, and gradually lower in the evening to facilitate restful sleep.

The decrease in cortisol in the evening is designed to ensure our body gets the signal that it is time for sleep.

This is when the cascade of neurotransmitters, hormones, and body temperature changes that occur prior to sleep, all come to play and your body prepares for a good night of shut-eye!

Come morning, the curve illustrates how cortisol starts to escalate from the early hours of the morning until it eventually brings us out of sleep to start our day, and so begins the morning half of the bell curve – a spike in cortisol!

The rise in cortisol throughout the morning is what gives us energy, increases our heart rate slightly, liberates stored energy, dumps those energy stores into the bloodstream to burn as fuel, and gets us geared up to tackle the world!

This cortisol spike then reaches its peak around late morning to midday, and then begins its natural descent into the decline we spoke of above, completing the diurnal curve nicely!

It goes up and down on this beautifully orchestrated hormonal symphony, regulating our metabolism, energy production, cognitive function, and nervous system as we navigate night and day in this wonderful thing, we call life!

CORTISOL AND THE STRESS RESPONSE

Now outside of this normal curve where cortisol follows its natural rhythms, the other functions of this hormone shine brightest when stressful situations arise.

These stressors may be real, imagined, physical, or emotional in nature, but all have the same affect. When someone confronts a situation, the brain deems it a risk or a danger, our senses send the alarm bell to the amygdala, an area in the basal region of the brain.

The amygdala is an old architecture responsible for governing not just emotional processing, but also gut instinct, fear, intuition, and survival instincts.

The amygdala interprets the images and sounds from our eyes and ears when it perceives the situation to be a threat or that we are in danger. Upon determining if a situation is life or death, it instantly sends a distress signal to the hypothalamus.

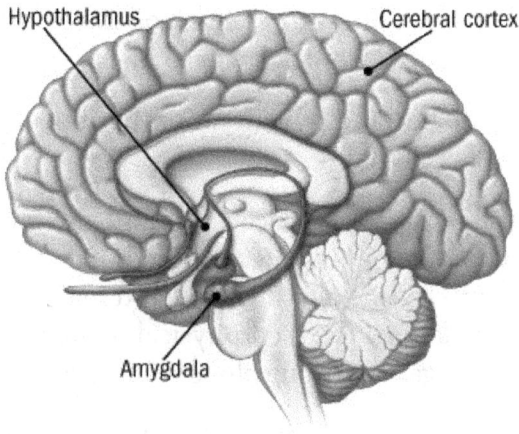

Figure 2A – The regions of the brain that initiate the stress response

The hypothalamus will then ensure that the body will treat this stressful event as its highest priority, ensuring the survival of the host as its main priority!

It will start a complex symphony of stress hormone physiology.

The hypothalamus will send signals to the adrenal glands, that sit atop the kidneys, to release adrenaline and cortisol.

Simultaneously, Norepinephrine, a stimulatory neurotransmitter that will heighten blood flow to the brain, is increased in the brain, and will ensure you have razor-sharp focus for the task at hand.

Once the adrenal glands get the word from the hypothalamus, they will send out a surge of adrenaline to boot us into flight-or-fight mode, alongside cortisol.

These hormones will increase blood flow to the extremities to ensure that our muscles have plenty of oxygen, whilst also stimulating (through glucagon) the release of stored muscle glycogen into the blood to get quick sugar to burn.

It changes our focus, and our attention becomes narrowed to the immediate task at hand.

Adrenaline will increase your heart rate and also increase blood pressure as cortisol manipulates the sodium regulating hormone aldosterone to thicken the blood and make more electrolytic salts available for increased physical demand. It also continues to dump sugar into your blood for quick fuel.

Our palms get clammy, our breath becomes shallower, and we tend to breathe faster and from the chest, as opposed to deep breaths from the diaphragm as you would expect in a calm and well-rested person's respiration.

By this stage in the stress response, we have well and truly put ourselves in a strong position to deal with whatever situation is at hand.

We have ample fuel to burn, with adrenaline and cortisol flowing through our system driving blood to the large muscle groups to get us ready to either punch or run, and we have tunnel vision focus on whatever is in our immediate path.

You are essentially switching into 'sports mode' to use a car analogy.

You have well and truly engaged the overdrive and are primed physically and mentally to take on any task at hand! Your body has you in peak performance mode to ensure that if you need to get out of a stressful situation to survive, you can do so!

The craziest part of the above stress response is that all of these changes happen so quickly that people aren't aware of them.

It is practically instantaneous!

This stress response circuitry is so efficient and well ingrained into our biology that the amygdala and hypothalamus kick-start this hormonal cascade even before the brain's visual centres have had a chance to fully process what is happening.

In layman's terms, you have already switched on 'sports mode' well before your body has had a chance to realise it is even stressing out!

This instantaneous stress response happens in the body because the nervous system can't afford to wait to see if a situation is life or death before acting.

Your survival wiring figures that are waiting to see if it is life or death may well cost you your life, so it punches first and asks questions later.

This innate and largely invisible stress response is why people are able to make extraordinary physical feats like jump out of the path of an oncoming car, even before they think about what they are doing.

The body has already done all of this work in the background to ensure you were primed to get out of harm's way, well and truly before your body registers the physical feeling of the stress physiology cascade!

This state of being is referred to as being in the sympathetic state of our nervous system.

Sympathetic states are associated with having the accelerator on, well and truly, as we described above. This state is essential for survival and is what we activate whenever our nervous system interprets the environment as having a situation requiring us to be in this state to tackle the task at hand.

THE PARASYMPATHETIC NERVOUS SYSTEM – THE BODY'S HANDBRAKE TO STRESS RESPONSES

It is a fact of life that what goes up must come down.

The stress response is no exception to this law.

This dance of the sympathetic nervous system and what we call the HPA axis (hypothalamus, pituitary-adrenal axis) with its complex hormonal symphony is well and truly the 'up' we speak of here.

Being in flight-or-fight mode means our nervous system has been jacked up, to deal with life-threatening or stressful situations.

This is where the fundamental truth from above comes into play, being so 'up' and wired definitely has a balancing system in the body to ensure we also come down.

So how does this specifically play out?

If 'up' is flight-or-fight mode, with your entire body primed to either punch or run, then what does 'down' look like?

Down starts with the tipping of the balancing beam, so to speak, for your nervous system.

After the stress response has done its job and hopefully gotten us out of harm's way, then we engage what we call the parasympathetic nervous system (PNS).

The easiest way to describe the functions of the PNS is to think of them as 'rest-and-digest' as opposed to 'flight-or-fight'.

The PNS is all about stimulating repair, recovery, digestion, and returning our body to homeostasis. We will cover this in greater depth shortly.

But in layman's terms, the body starts putting on the brakes to wind us down and return to normal physiology and recover from whatever the hell we just tackled!

Our cortisol starts winding back down to baseline levels and continues to follow the diurnal curve we saw in Figure 1, and our adrenaline decreases. Epinephrine and other stimulating neurotransmitters in the brain decline to the baseline levels.

Breath rate slows and deepens, blood supply to working muscles returns to normal, our heart rate decreases, and our blood pressure returns to normal.

All of the stimulatory systems of the HPA axis's response to stress begin to wind down, and the parasympathetic system starts to switch gears into recovery mode.

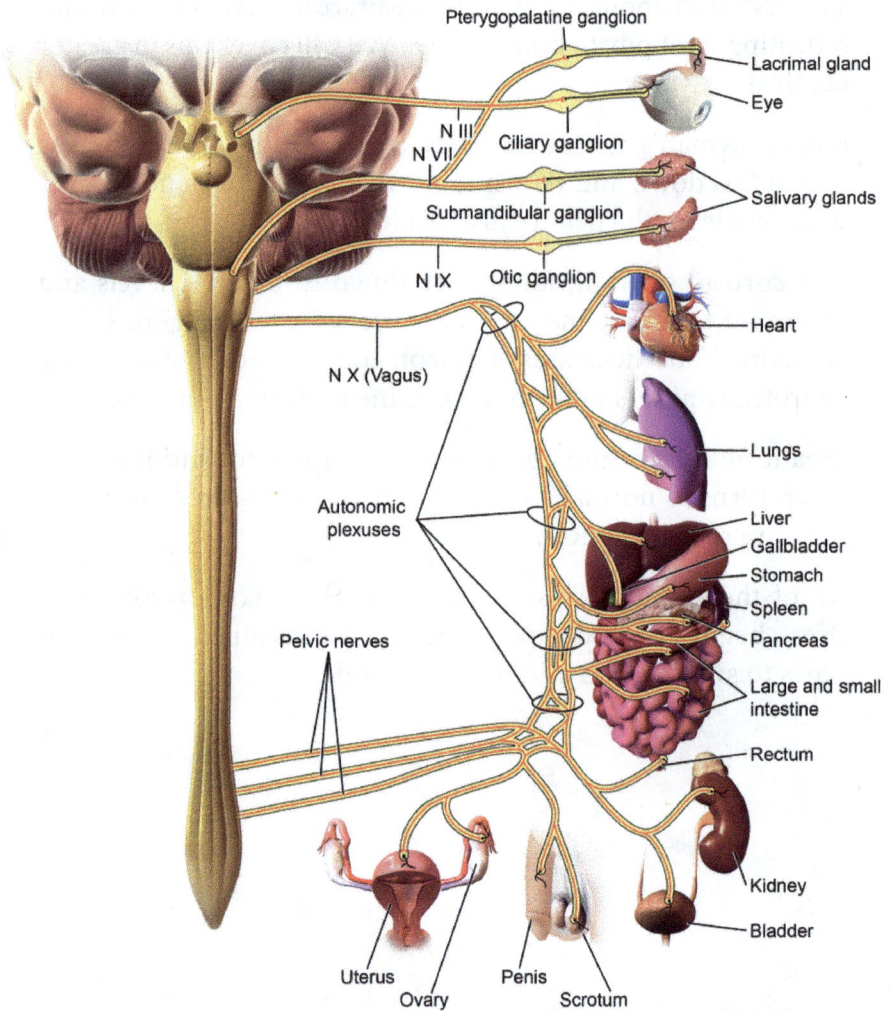

Parasympathetic Innervation

Figure 3A – The parasympathetic nervous system and how it interacts with every major system via nerve innovation

As seen in Figure 3A, just like the sympathetic nervous system interacts with every major system, so does the handbrake system of the parasympathetic.

The nervous system is a complex system of nerves that connects the brain with every cell of every organ of every tissue in the body.

Picture it like a superhighway that works off electrical impulses that travel from the brain, down these highways (nerves) to carry the message of what is required of each of the systems of the body (1).

The Parasympathetic Nervous System (PNS) is powerful at promoting repair, recovery, digestion, hormone production, and regulating homeostasis.

It allows the body to return to normal after enduring a stress response. In that process, allows much of the reversal of the flight-or-fight mode, and is a potent regulator of all systems coming back to baseline to be rebuilt and repaired.

The PNS and the SNS are the Yin and Yang of the stress response.

SNS is the up and PNS is the down. The accelerator and the handbrake, respectively.

Flight-or-fight versus rest-and-digest.

The activation of these two spheres of our nervous system will dictate much of our long-term health and particularly, how long we spend in each part of our nervous system will greatly dictate long-term health outcomes.

SO HOW DOES THIS GO WRONG?

The body's stress response is a well-oiled machine that will always be prioritised over every other biological function to ensure survival of the host.

No matter what other biological function we are referring to, whether the body has a full laundry list of jobs around metabolism, immune function, or hormone production to get done, once the stress response alarm sounds, it will cause a worker's strike from all of these other duties, so as to focus solely on surviving this immediate threat to our safety.

Now, what is worthy of mention here is that whilst the laundry list may get delayed whilst the body is dealing with the survival situation, it will still get tended to in short order, because in caveman times we would only have the odd life or death situation arise that we have to sporadically deal with, before we could carry on our merry way and resume normal biological functions.

Stress responses used to be isolated incidents in our evolutionary history, so this wasn't such a biggie.

As hunter-gatherers, your HPA axis was your guardian angel because every threat was likely actually life-threatening in early human history.

As cavemen, it could be due to freezing cold, going days without food, being attacked by wild animals, or being bitten by something venomous.

These were singular but very real dangers that the early human species faced.

The stress response physiology would be called upon in these times and get us out of harm's way. It was a superstar that kept us alive in hard times and was able to take on a harsh world full of unknown life-and-death encounters!

Now these stressors may be more life-threatening in our caveman lifestyles than in modern times, after all we are no longer being chased by sabretooth tigers or hunting mammoths with spears!

Back then, we would have our stress response play out, and we would engage our fight-or-flight mode to combat the sabretooth or spear the mammoth, get ourselves to safety, and then get on with the job of living.

The whole stress physiology response would then settle down to normal and resume the diurnal curve we spoke of, illustrated in Figure 3 below. We would be able to go back to our laundry list of biological chores and carry on with our day!

Daily Free Cortisol with Cortisol Awakening Response

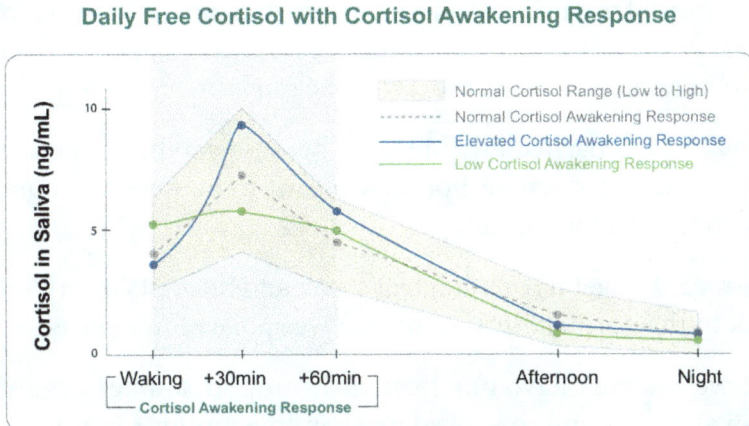

Figure 4 – Elevated Waking cortisol responses shown during stressful events. The Blue line indicates how cortisol escalates in response to stressors and in presence of chronic stress will often result in a strong surge in the morning cortisol.

Figure 3 here, demonstrates what this may have looked like in early human times when our survival systems evolved. Whilst this diagram is all about the CAR, what it shows is how after a stressor, cortisol still eventually gets back to its normal curve.

The spike is noted around the 30-minute mark that lasts for an hour approximately, before declining into the normal levels you would expect to see in the curve.

SO WHEN DO THE WHEELS FEEL OFF?

We can see that our body knows exactly what to do in response to a stressor.

It boots its stress hormones out to prime the body to deal with the threat, before returning to normality of the diurnal rhythm later in the day.

But the tricky part is that the curse of modern living is jam-packed with stressful responses. It is a laden with stressors, be it psychological, financial, emotional, imagined, or anticipated; there are dozens of sources of stress in the day of the modern man.

Now, this is a particularly big issue because you have to understand that this stress response is meant to be here for a good time but not a long time.

It is meant to get us out of harm's way and be on its merry way, back to the normal diurnal rhythm we spoke of in Figure 1.

But we humans have our lives drowning in sources of stress from all angles and so we end up spending our lives in this state of chronically elevated cortisol and stress.

Figure 3 demonstrates this perfectly.

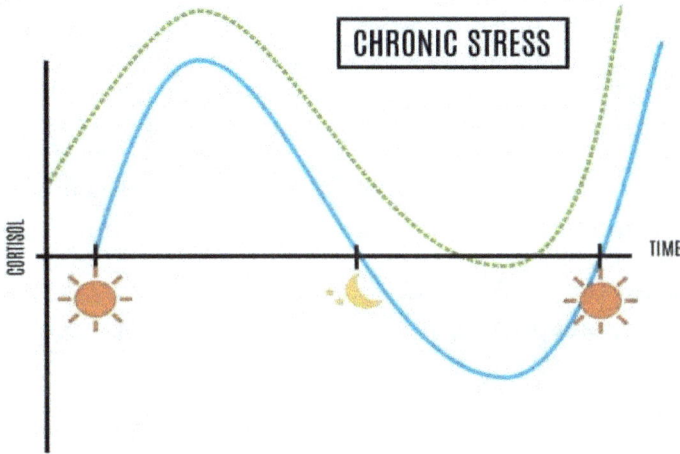

Figure 5 – The demonstration of modern living and its implications on cortisol. Chronic stress elevates baseline cortisol levels leading to a host of negative implications.

This is where I most commonly come across people at my seminars and workshops. This is where most people spend most of their lives. In a state of constant stress response.

A state of anxiety, angst, and being in constant flight-or-fight, and the sad part is it's so normal now, that people don't even realise they are living on adrenaline and cortisol most of their days!

Stress physiology was never designed to be elevated for a long term.

We have evolved to have this system as our back up in case of wild times where it would be engaged, then as quickly as it came, be disengaged.

And this is why the wheels fall off with people now in modern society.

The chronic state of being in a permanent stress response is biologically cooking people without anyone even realising it!

And sadly, there is a price to pay for living in crisis mode for a long term, a price that many are starting to pay, unfortunately.

The 2022 study (1A) by Chu et al. describes a stress response and the maladaptive risk when it is chronically present in our lives:

'*Any physical or psychological stimuli that disrupts homeostasis result in a stress response. The stimuli are called stressors and physiological and behavioural changes in response to exposure to stressors constitute the stress response. A stress response is mediated by a complex interplay of nervous, endocrine, and immune mechanisms that involves activation of the sympathetic-adreno-medullar (SAM) axis, the hypothalamus-pituitary-adrenal (HPA) axis, and immune system. The stress response is adaptive, to begin with, that prepares the body to handle the challenges presented by an internal or external environmental challenge (stressor)... But if the exposure to a stressor is actually or perceived as intense, repetitive (repeated acute stress), or prolonged (chronic stress), the stress response becomes maladaptive and detrimental to physiology e.g., exposure to chronic stressors can cause maladaptive reactions including depression, anxiety, cognitive impairment, and heart disease.*'

We are inundated with stimuli that our body deems as stressors on the daily.

This leads to chronic elevation of cortisol, and our stress physiology which then leads down to the path of a host of metabolic diseases, inflammation, gut issues like leaky gut and IBS, hormonal imbalances in women, low testosterone in men, holding of stubborn fat, wasting of muscle mass, anxiety, depression, and compromised immune function.

The body was only meant to use the sympathetic nervous system's stress response as a 'break glass in case of an emergency' scenario. Modern man is unfortunately setting off this metaphorical fire alarm 20 times a day, and we then wonder why when we look at society so many people are experiencing increases in inflammation, gut issues, hormonal diseases, metabolic issues, infertility, and depression?!

The writing is on the wall, medically speaking.

Modern society is one big walking cortisol symptom picture.

The signs and symptoms of chronic stress responses are everywhere, screaming at an audience of deaf ears, who themselves are swimming in an ocean of cortisol and angst.

The pace at which we live life is well and truly at odds with how our physiology was designed.

We were never made to have near-constant engagement of our flight-or-fight systems and to have our HPA axis on overdrive.

SO WHAT ARE THE SYMPTOM PICTURES OF CHRONICALLY ELEVATED CORTISOL?

A better heading for this section of the book may as well have been 'A Description of the Modern Condition'.

By the end of this checklist, you will likely be left feeling 'triggered' after ticking 90% of it that we are about to rattle off.

So, do the author a favour. Come with me now and perform a mental audit of your own daily life, and see if you experience any of the following symptomology in your day, week, or month.

1. Feeling Tired but Wired
2. Taking a Long Time to get to Sleep
3. Poor Sleep Quality
4. Anxiety, Depression, Angst, and Low Mood
5. Stubborn Body Fat Around the Lower Stomach and High Visceral Fat
6. Low Testosterone in Men
7. Hormonal Imbalances in Women Including Disruption of Monthly Cycle
8. High Blood Pressure
9. Elevated Resting Heart Rate
10. Low Libido
11. Slowing of Metabolic Rate (Looking at Food and Putting on Weight)
12. Fluid Retention, Looking Swollen and Puffy
13. Poor Immune System Function
14. Poor Blood Sugar Control and Craving Sugary and Fatty Foods

KNOW THY ENEMY – 'STRESS' VS STRESSORS

Throughout this book, you will see the word 'stress' hundreds of times.

But for the purpose of this book, it is worthy of note that most people's relationship with stress needs some expansion in its definitions and understanding.

The average person, when asked the simple question:

'How much stress is in your life currently?'

Will scan their conscious mind for anxiety and mentally perceived stress in the present moment.

This is their entire assessment, whether they are feeling anxious, or stressed in this current moment when asked the question.

Upon concluding that they are probably handling themselves okay today, they will then reply:

'Nothing really major. I am pretty chill. I don't have a lot of stress in my day.'

However, as we have learned above, this is where the great logic fallacy occurs!

The stress response, as we covered earlier in the book, is instantaneous in the face of perceived threats.

It is literally kicking in before you have even realised you are stressing.

So, when people are doing a personal assessment of their stress levels, it has two problems.

One is that anxiety, angst, and perceived stress is merely one symptom of high stress hormones, and not necessarily the best indicator of the amount of stress on the body at any point in time.

Second, is the fact that even if you were accurate in pinpointing that you are currently stressed, your stress response has already beat you to the finish line, and your perception of your own stress is likely very late to the party.

In layman's terms, you're stressed and you don't even know it!

So, now that we have identified the two major issues with how people assess their own stress levels, it is important to take an overview of your life to get a grasp on the true extent and presence of stress!

In our lives, we must expand our understanding of what stress actually is and how many areas it can come from!

We must also accept that, as we covered earlier, the problem with self-identifying one's level of stress is that the actual physical stress response is instantaneous.

The sympathetic nervous system and its flight-or-fight stress response is engaged literally even before your senses register it happening.

You are literally red lining, ready to take on the perceived threat before your body has had time to register it!

So you can see how it is problematic to rely on your own analysis of how much time you spend in flight-or-fight when it kicks in literally faster than your senses register it!

Elizabeth Scott, PhD, is an author, workshop leader, educator, and award-winning blogger on stress management, positive psychology, relationships, and emotional well-being.

Her definition of Stress is as follows:

'Stress can be defined as any type of change that causes physical, emotional, or psychological strain. Stress is your body's response to anything that requires attention or action.'

Any type of change that requires attention or action.

This is a far more comprehensive overview of stress and is in direct opposition to the very limiting and commonly accepted definition of stress by organisations such as the World Health Organization that defines stress as simply *a state of worry or mental tension caused by a difficult situation'*.

So when we talk about stress in this book, we will be talking about 'stressors', which will include a large list of stimuli that can cause change and require immediate attention and action by the body, thus categorising it as stress, as per our definition above.

So, for the purpose of clarifying all the sources of stressors that one may be experiencing in their life, I have compiled a more holistic list below to use as a checklist. As an exercise now, on a spare piece of paper, create a checklist.

Do an audit of your current lifestyle and write down any of the following listed stressors that may appear in your day, week, month, or year.

If you have found that your list includes multiple sources from this list, it is safe to assume your body is undergoing some degree of stress, whether you recognise it as the symptom of having anxiety or mentally perceived stress, or not!

In fact, a great exercise here is to look at your checklist of all the stressors that may be present in your life from this list, and note the lack of actual mentally perceived stress in your conscious right now!

This will directly demonstrate that your body has an abundance of stressors, and is therefore 'stressed', even if mentally you have zero registers of it in the form of perceived stress or anxiety!

AN AUDIT OF STRESSORS ON THE BODY:

- **Inflammation** – This can be from acute sources, such as injuries, sprains, tears, or more insidious and systemic, such as inflammation in our gut lining, or the presence of elevated inflammatory intermediary compounds in our body such as interleukin 6 (IL-6). Blood tests are often the only way we can easily recognise this more systemic inflammation by looking for the IL-6 or C-reactive protein. Not all inflammation is easily recognised or perceived!

- **Unresolved Emotional Trauma** – Whilst this book is more about the physical sources of stress, it is widely accepted (and thankfully promoted by progressive practitioners such as the world-renowned Canadian practitioner, psychologist, and author, Gabor Mate) that trauma during childhood and early developmental years directly influences the nervous system. Trauma and unresolved emotional tension can act out in the body by chronically increasing stress hormone output as well as increasing our stress response to a given stressor. This is a very subtle and often subconscious source of stress and something we will unpack later in more detail.

- **Alcohol Consumption** – Alcohol is a Catch-22 of sorts. Consumption of alcohol is known to increase the inhibitory neurotransmitter GABA. GABA is associated with feelings of calmness, well-being, and is directly antagonistic to adrenaline, norepinephrine, and cortisol, our primary stress hormones. So, on the one hand, it will acutely increase feelings of calmness and reduce perceived stress and anxiety. However, regular alcohol consumption increases stress by disrupting sleep quality. This is reinforced by dozens of studies, and echoed by the National Institute of Health statement: *'Prolonged Alcohol con-*

sumption is associated with chronic sleep disturbance, lower slow wave sleep, and more rapid eye movement sleep than normal'. It has also been demonstrated in recent research by neuroscientist Dr. Andrew Huberman from Stanford University, that alcohol consumption increased stress response to a given stressor when consumed regularly. So, in the immediate experience alcohol decreases the perception of stress, but immediately after this it will directly increase stress by impairing sleep quality and increasing stress hormone output to a given stressor.

This relationship is summarised perfectly by an excerpt from the study 'Alcohol, Aging, and the Stress Response' conducted by Robert L. Spencer, PhD, and Kent E. Hutchison, PhD, in the *Alcohol Research and Health* journal of the National Institute of Health:

'The body responds to stress through a hormone system called the hypothalamic-pituitary adrenal (HPA) axis. Stimulation of this system results in the secretion of stress hormones (i.e., glucocorticoids). Chronic excessive glucocorticoid secretion can have adverse health effects, such as Cushing's syndrome. Alcohol intoxication activates the HPA axis and results in elevated glucocorticoid levels. Ironically, elevated levels of these stress hormones may contribute to alcohol's pleasurable effects. With chronic alcohol consumption, however, tolerance may develop to alcohol's HPA axis-activating effects. Chronic alcohol consumption, as well as chronic glucocorticoid exposure, can result in premature and/or exaggerated aging. Furthermore, the aging process affects a person's sensitivity to alcohol and HPA axis function. Thus, a three-way interaction exists among alcohol consumption, HPA axis activity, and the aging process. The aging process may impair the HPA axis' ability to adapt to

chronic alcohol exposure. Furthermore, HPA axis activation may contribute to the premature or exaggerated aging associated with chronic alcohol consumption.' (1)

Sleep will be covered far more extensively in later chapters of this book, but in short, there is a very clear loop that exists. High stressors lead to poor sleep quality. Poor sleep quality leads to higher levels of stress hormones. Around and around the circuit goes!

- **Relationship strain or breakdown** – This is the most self-explanatory of the sources of stress on the body in this list thus far. Relationship issues are a massive and common source of stress in modern lives. Maintaining a healthy relationship in the face of the increased cost of living, working hours, and the increasing pace of modern life is a big task and often results in its fair share of emotional strain. Emotional stress is no different from physical sources of stress in the chemistry of our stress response.
- **Poor Gut Health** – The gut and stress share a two-way relationship. Stress inflames the gut lining via the effects of the protein zonulin, whilst also increasing inflammatory markers such as interleukin 6.

This relationship showing how stress immediately affects inflammation was demonstrated perfectly in the study by Linninge et al. in 2018:

'This study aimed to examine gut permeability and physiological and inflammatory markers of reactivity to acute psychosocial stress. Forty young men were classified as high-stressed (HIGHS) or low-stressed (LOWS) according to the Shirom-Melamed Burnout Questionnaire. Cardiovascular reactivity and gut dysfunction were studied along with cortisol, zonulin and

cytokines. Gut permeability was shown to be affected within one hour after the psychosocial stress induction... Interleukin-6 increased with time, most pronounced at the end of the one-hour recovery after V-TSST...HIGHS experienced more abdominal dysfunction compared to LOWS. In conclusion, this study is the first to show fluctuations in gut permeability after psychosocial stress induction. This was partly associated with changes in inflammatory markers.'

Inversely, the inflammatory compounds released by an inflamed gut lining also drive stress in the body! This creates a vicious loop whereby stress inflames the gut and an inflamed gut causes stress.

- **Poor Sleep Quality** – Poor sleep directly correlates with increased stress levels. This is demonstrated in the 2015 study from the Institute of Sleep Science by Hirotsu C. et al.:

'Poor sleep quality due to sleep disorders and sleep loss is highly prevalent in the modern society. Underlying mechanisms show that stress is involved in the relationship between sleep and metabolism through hypothalamic-pituitary-adrenal (HPA) axis activation. Sleep deprivation and sleep disorders are associated with maladaptive changes in the HPA axis, leading to neuroendocrine dysregulation. Excess of glucocorticoids increase glucose and insulin and decrease adiponectin levels. Thus, this review provides overall view of the relationship between sleep, stress, and metabolism from basic physiology to pathological conditions, highlighting effective treatments for metabolic disturbances.' (2)

Sleep is such a crucial player in stress and stress hormone secretion that we will cover this in much greater detail in later chapters of this book. For the time being, just understand that the most protective thing we have against chronic stress is a deep, refreshing sleep!

- **Over-caffeination** – The relationship of caffeine and cortisol is best covered in this study excerpt:

'Caffeine also activates the stress axis, elevating glucocorticoid and catecholamine output along with increases in blood pressure. As such, caffeine intake during times of stress may contribute to the duration and magnitude of blood pressure and stress endocrine responses.' (3) (4)

This relationship of caffeine consumption and cortisol is acute and lasting, as observed in the study above (4).

The figure below (Fig. 1) is extracted from this study and demonstrates the immediate spike in cortisol after caffeine consumption. It also shows that it takes approximately 3 hours for the cortisol to decline post-consumption. Here, caffeine was administered at 9 am, 1 pm, and 6 pm. You can plainly see that at every ingestion of caffeine there is a transitory spike in cortisol!

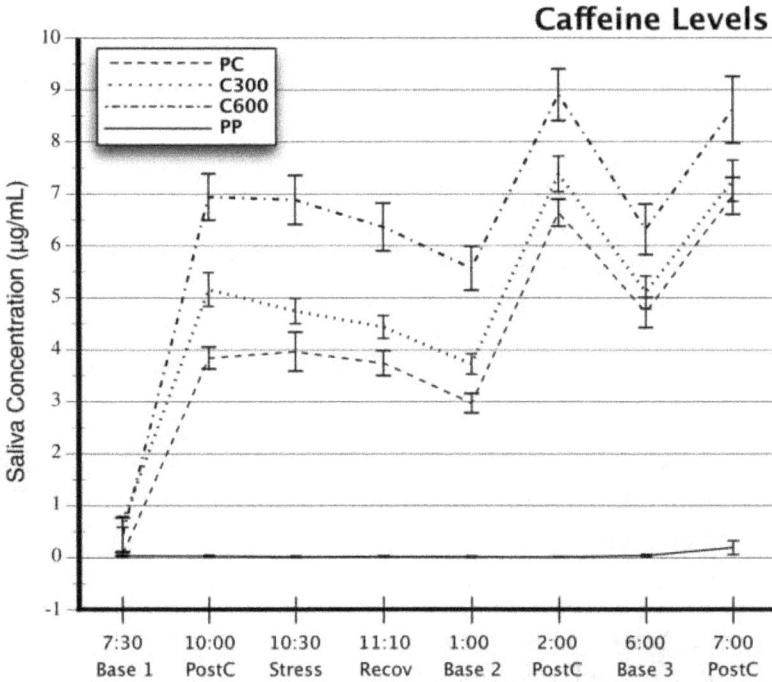

Figure 6 – Caffeine concentrations in saliva on 4 test days. Entries show means and error bars that represent standard errors. Samples from 7:30 am to 2:00 pm were collected in the laboratory and the samples at 6:00 and 7:00 pm were collected at home. PC = placebo caffeine concentrations in saliva on 4 test days. Entries show means, and error bars represent standard errors. Samples from 7:30 am to 2:00 pm were collected in the laboratory, and the samples at 6:00 and 7:00 pm were collected at home. PC = placebo maintenance followed by 3 × 250 mg caffeine challenges on the test day. C300 = 300 mg/day of caffeine at home followed by caffeine challenge on the test day. C600 = 600 mg/day at home followed by caffeine challenge on the test day. PP = placebo at home and placebo on test day. Base 1, Base 2, Base 3 = saliva samples taken immediately before taking a caffeine or placebo capsule. PostC = samples taken 1 hour postdrug. Stress and Recov = samples taken at the end of a 30-minute behavioural stress period or after 30 minutes of recovery.

To look closer at how much this caffeine consumption affected cortisol, we looked at another study which demonstrated:

'Following caffeine (consumption), ACTH was significantly elevated at all times from 30 min to 180 min, and CORT was elevated from 60 min to 120 min. Peak increases relative to placebo were: ACTH, 33% (+5.2 pg/ml) and CORT, 30% (+2.7 micrograms/dl) at 60 min post caffeine.' (5)

In short, after ingesting caffeine, cortisol and the associated hormone ACTH were increased, from nearly immediately after consumption to well over 3 hours later.

A 30% increase in cortisol is a very significant increase in stress for the body!

Keeping caffeine consumption below 300 mg per day would be a recommendation of this author, as even at 300 mg of caffeine daily, split evenly into 3 doses of 100 mg each, this was still a very significant increase in stress on the body!

- **Financial Stress** – With cost of living at an all-time high, the average level of debt in Australia at its historical peak, it is no wonder that people are stressed by money!
- **Excessive Mental Stimulus** – With the frantic pace with which we live the modern life, it is no wonder that stress is a common phenomenon for the everyday Joe! Now mental stimulation can be multi-factorial, it is the result of time spent on smartphones, tablets, and laptops, filling every possible second of the day with something that requires focus. Take an audit of your day from the minute you get up to the minute you go to bed. I can guarantee, every moment of potential downtime has been filled with some sort of stimulus. Particularly, in the form of scrolling on social media platforms. The times when we would have historically had time for our brains to rest and for us

to have quiet time has been filled in entirety with smart-phones, Netflix, and DMs!

This constant state of having to be mentally switched on will directly affect your nervous system's ability to slip into 'rest-and-digest', also known as the parasympathetic element of your nervous system. Taking time to actually let your cognitive load decline is a potent antidote for a common source of stress!

- **Shift Work** – This is a fascinating topic and one that impacts massive portions of the population.

According to the Australian Bureau of Statistics, a 2009 survey showed that 16% of the entire Australian workforce engaged in shift work (6). That is a huge portion of the workforce who are spending the majority of their weeks awake when they were bio-logically designed to be asleep!

The implications of shift work have become an area of consider-able interest and are a massive source of stress for the body.

Firstly, shift work was demonstrated to lead to an increased inflammation in the body.

We have made mention of markers of elevated inflammation in the body previously with the two compounds, C-reactive pro-tein and interleukin 6.

This study demonstrated that shift work was demonstrated to increase both of these inflammatory compounds via its disrup-tion of sleep and circadian rhythm:

'Shift work is closely related to sleep deprivation and disturbance, causing immune dysfunction as elevated concentrations of C-reactive protein and interleukin 6, and an increase in cellular stress in terms

of an altered balance of pro-oxidative and anti-oxidative markers'
(7).

Now, inflammation is in itself a common source of stress in the body. But to further this study, cortisol was directly measured in shift workers to see if this pattern of work was related to increases in stress hormones:

'Using urinary or hair cortisol, two studies from the US and the Netherlands respectively observed that shift workers had significantly higher cortisol levels. Also, a British study showed that shift work was associated with higher waking cortisol as well as total AUC in saliva'
(8, 9, 10).

This was furthered by the findings of the 2018 study that looked at 1000 German physicians who participated in shift work. The results of this study concluded the following:

'The aim of our study was to examine the longitudinal impact of shift work on diurnal cortisol rhythm. Drawing on a sample of junior physicians from Germany, we found that shift work at baseline significantly changed the diurnal cortisol pattern at follow-up, in terms of higher waking cortisol, steeper slope and larger AUC, thereby predicting increased cortisol secretion at follow-up' *(11).*

The waking cortisol was also examined in the 2018 study, as is seen in Figure 2 below.

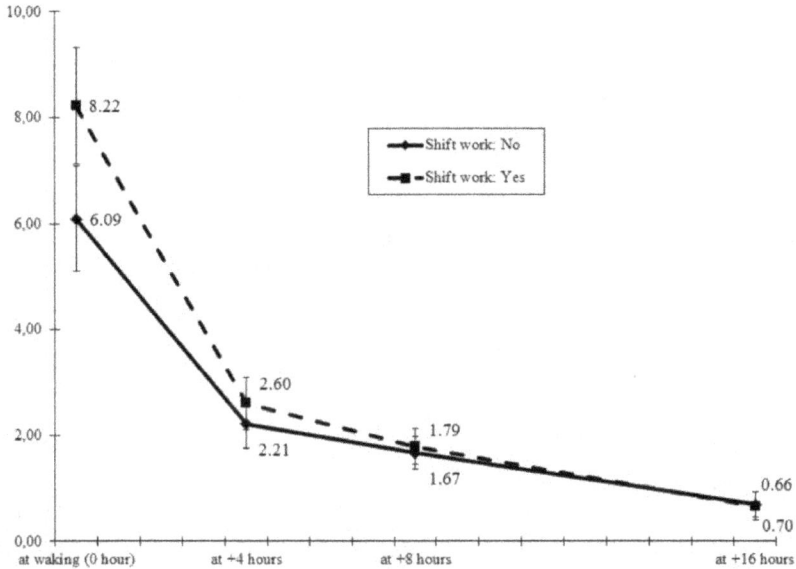

Figure 7 – illustrates diurnal cortisol rhythm at follow-up for the shift work group vs. the non-shift work group.

Figure 2 shows a 26% increase in waking cortisol levels upon waking in shift workers vs non-shift workers (8.22 vs 6.09).

All in all, it is clear in the data that shift work is very much shifting the fundamental biological rhythms of our body. This is in turn leading to long-term increases in stress hormones and inflammation in the body and is a powerful contributor to stress burden if you are unlucky enough to have this rostering arrangement!

- **Nutrient Deficiencies** – This is another interesting source of stress and is in itself a negative feedback loop system. That is to say that nutrient deficiencies are shown to increase stress on the body and stress also leads to micro-nutrient deficiencies!

In fact, most clear data is showing the lowering effects stress has on micronutrients. There were hundreds of reputable studies showing this link between high cortisol and depletion of valuable micronutrients.

So, for the purpose of this source of stress, it has been clearly demonstrated that lower concentrations of magnesium, zinc, vitamin C, and vitamin D can cause increases in stress (11,12). But what was also interesting to explore was the relationship between stress and how it then further lowers those vitamins.

The Holtorf Medical Group summarised it perfectly with this excerpt:

'The adrenals are an important part of the endocrine system as they are two little glands that sit on the top of the kidneys that both produce and regulate the stress hormone cortisol. The adrenal glands also produce sex hormones, estrogen and progesterone, neurotransmitters, adrenaline (epinephrine), norepinephrine, and dopamine. These hormones and neurotransmitters regulate the metabolism and communicate with other organs such as the brain, kidneys, and reproductive system.

Thus, when the body is lacking the nutrients required for proper adrenal function, your health can quickly become compromised.'

To make this even easier to conceptualise, imagine the analogy when you are in flight-or-fight mode (i.e., experiencing high cortisol), you will find that it is like you are driving a car around in sports mode.

You feel like you're flying, living on adrenaline and cortisol, and so are 'ON' and wired.

But you also burn a lot of fuel and resources when in 'sports mode'.

Some of those resources that you burn at the rapid rate we are describing in this analogy are micronutrients, in particular, vitamins B1,2,6,12, magnesium, zinc and vitamin C (12).

This is summarised perfectly in the 2020 study from the Lopresti et al.:

'Excess or chronic psychological or environmental stress is associated with an increased risk of mental and physical diseases, with several mechanisms theorised to be associated with its detrimental effects. One underappreciated potential mechanism relates to the effects of psychological and environmental stress on micronutrient concentrations. Micronutrients (vitamins and minerals) are essential for optimal physical and mental function, with deficiencies associated with an array of diseases' (12).

The 2020 meta-analysis (12) referenced above, demonstrated perfectly in a range of situations how both acute and chronic stress affected the micronutrients magnesium, zinc, calcium, iron, and the B vitamins.

In addition, stress was also demonstrated to deplete electrolytes (13), sodium, potassium, magnesium, and calcium:

'In conclusion, the result of this study suggest that alteration of serum electrolyte caused by repeated restrained in water-treated and ethanol-treated rats could possibly occur due to an increase in sympathetic activity leading to enhanced excretion of these electrolytes.'

In this study, they applied stressors to rats and measured the electrolyte status and found serum levels declined after stress tests.

This was also the case with the 2020 study above, which analysed over 50 research papers on stress and its effects on various nutrients and found that stress acutely and chronically affected micronutrient levels.

Micronutrients are definitely the foundations of our biology, and the ones listed in the meta-analysis are crucial for hormone production, energy production, nervous system regulation, and brain health.

So, it is clear to see why chronic stress would affect so many systems in the body and how there is a two-way relationship between micronutrient deficiency and stress, as well as stress and associated nutrient deficiencies!

- **Undereating (Accidentally or on Purpose) and Dieting**

The world we live in now is a very superficial, body conscious one.

Whilst one could argue, this social media-driven Vanity Fair is beneficial (considering two-thirds of the population of the USA is now considered overweight, with one-third of that being clinically classed as obese) (14A), it definitely has led to a very clear trend!

General population (gen pop, as the fitness industry refers to them) has become obsessed with losing weight on a large scale!

This is on a much wider scale than even this author realised. When researching for this section of the book, I came across the startling 2005 statistic that indicated that approximately 47% of adults in the United States are trying to lose weight at any given time (14B).

That was 18 years ago at the time of writing this book as well! That was only the early era of social media-driven body obsession and dieting culture truly going boom! I could only imagine that in present times this would be the vast majority of people! Dieting and fat loss have forged entire industries.

Now, before I tie this into the take-home message, dieting is technically a great thing! As a long-term member of the fitness industry, I have personally helped countless people to diet successfully and lose weight in a healthy and sustainable way.

This is a great mission statement as well!

Helping a sedentary population losing a few kilos over the summer is almost always great for overall health.

However, the 'but' comes in when people diet without guidance or any nutritional literacy themselves and often end up grossly undereating. They are, in many cases, also undereating already so when they put themselves in a deliberate calorie deficit, their body freaks out! It can be likened to an overworked and understaffed corporate department. The department is already running on minimal resources, doing the best they can with what meagre capital (think calories) they have! Then head office really puts the boot in and institutes more budget cuts!

This is so typical of many of the gen pop clients I have crossed paths with. Many of them are busy-working folk, or overworked parents, and they typically start the day skipping breakfast in favour of a coffee. Caffeine, we have already established, is in itself a stimulant that increases cortisol.

Then lunch is something (usually of low nutritional value) they can grab on the run, maybe a sandwich or a wrap. Or even more commonly, this is substituted for a take away muffin with their third skim cappuccino for the day!

Dinner is meat and three veggies (if we are lucky and it's not from a drive-through on the way home). This day would be very low in total calories, high in total caffeine, and a perfect illustration of our understaffed corporate body analogy.

Having done this exercise with hundreds of people, personally I can say from anecdotal data that this is the norm for so many people, and more alarmingly these are the people who most likely make up 47% of the population wanting to lose weight at any given time.

So, you are chronically undereating, which in itself is a great way to impact thyroid function and slow down your metabolism. Then you throw in a bucket of coffee per day, again jacking up cortisol, and throwing fuel on the fire, biologically speaking. Then, Monday rolls around and we decide that today is day one of going on an aggressive keto diet!

The stress skyrockets on the body, and feeling lousy with the even further drop in calories, we turn to our old friend to get us through – caffeine!

We swap actual calories for liquid adrenaline, with our daily coffee becoming three double shot oat lattes by midday. We must push through the dieting brain fog at all costs!

The impact of this worked example of dieting on cortisol and thus stress on the body is so pronounced that there was a paper published on it literally named 'Low Calorie Dieting Increases Cortisol' (15).

An excerpt from the results section of this paper, pointed out perfectly how dieting can be a common source of stress for people:

'Restricting calories increased the total output of cortisol, and monitoring calories increased perceived stress. Conclusions: Dieting may be deleterious to psychological well-being and biological functioning, and changes in clinical recommendations may be in order... In addition, studies have found that higher dietary restraint (a measure of dieting) is associated with higher 24-hour urinary free cortisol concentrations, and cortisol-creatinine ratios, salivary cortisol, and cortisol awakening response'.

What this is highlighting is that dieting is a source of stress for many people just in and of itself. If I told you, reading along at home, that tomorrow morning we were starting an aggressive fat loss phase, I could damn near guarantee the cortisol spike!

So many people have a lot of emotional baggage, self-esteem, and self-worth tied up in historical attempts at modifying body composition. Weight loss magnifies this baggage and all the emotional associations of dieting come welling up to the surface as soon as we start the new meal plan.

This is one reason undereating is a common source of increased cortisol for a lot of people. Dieting itself is an unpleasant process and we associate it with other negative experiences around body image as soon as we start the fat loss phase. Reliably, stress goes up, and the data supports this!

Second reason undereating increases stress is because our system has a maintenance requirement. It has a number of calories it requires to maintain normal daily function, keeping your brain functioning, organs firing, and of course, getting those daily steps in!

Undereating means we are literally (whether on purpose or by accident) eating less than we need to function optimally.

This is an obviously stressful situation for the body when you look at it as a standalone statement.

You are eating less than your body needs to function. This is said a little more clearly in the 2010 study (14B):

'Restricting caloric intake may be a particularly salient biological stressor, because one of the main functions of cortisol is to increase the availability of energy in the body. The stress resulting from restricting one's caloric intake to a mere 1200 kcal, therefore, may have reduced the absolute amount of energy available to the body, leading to increased cortisol release energy stores.'

This is highlighted in this diagram from the 2010 study mentioned above, which demonstrates an increase in cortisol output as a result of dieting.

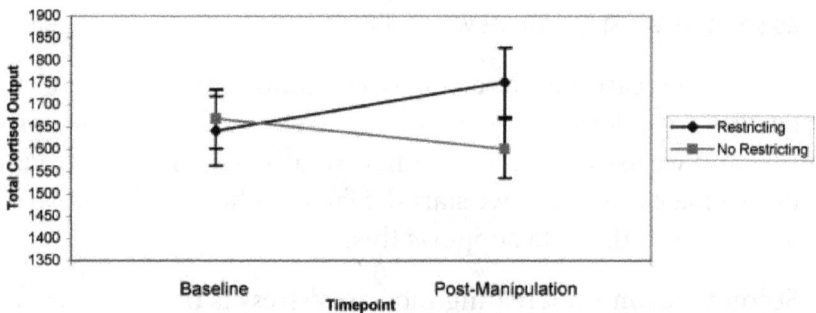

Figure 8 – Cortisol output comparing non-dieting (no restricting) with dieting (restricting) showing caloric restriction increased cortisol significantly.

SO HOW TO DIET WITHOUT PUTTING YOURSELF THROUGH HPA AXIS HELL?

Well, first and foremost, we need to do some housekeeping and point out an obvious fact.

The short-term pain of dieting doesn't negate the long-term benefits of carrying less body fat.

So, whilst being in a caloric deficit does temporarily increase stress on the body, it also is only a temporary and intentional exercise to reduce body fat and increase a host of health improving aspects of our biology in the process. When dieting is done correctly, the juice is worth the squeeze, and this author will not talk you out of losing those love handles!

What the issue with caloric restriction is that many who start diets are already undereating in the first place, and therefore are already experiencing high stress on the body. Their metabolism is also already underperforming from this chronic undereating and so they are starting the race with one leg tied. They are giving themselves almost zero chance of losing weight successfully and sustainably if they are already living on more caffeine than calories!

Undereating would have slowed their metabolism, making weight loss stubborn and unnecessarily stressful. The stress on their body from already undereating long-term would have also negatively impacted their basal metabolic rate (BMR) as well as through the known interactions of cortisol with the thyroid hormone reverse T3 (rT3). The increase of rT3 leads to a dampened BMR and any dieting attempts will be a very painful and slow process from here.

Instead, these folks who have been undereating should be encouraged to first tackle a phase of eating at their caloric maintenance to get themselves back to good metabolic health, and to lower cortisol, before attempting such diets.

The length of the maintenance phase will be dictated by the length of time the person has been in a caloric deficit, on purpose or otherwise.

So, if 40-year-old mother of 3, Susan, has been accidentally undereating and living on coffee for the last 2 years, it would be advised she spends a good 6 months at maintenance minimum to really restore homeostasis before attempting any further dieting.

This can be done through a steady 'reverse dieting' phase where we increase calories from current intake by 50–100 calories per week until maintenance calories are reached.

So, if Susan was accidentally only eating 1200 cal and her maintenance was say 1900, then it would take her approximately 2 months of adding 100 cal a week to get to her 1900 cal maintenance via reverse dieting. Then she will spend a good 6 months there to really repair the metabolic damage done by years of undereating. This may look like taking an entire year of purposely eating more food to get you into a much stronger place than when you started.

After the time spent at maintenance, Susan can start her dieting phase from 1900 cal as her regular intake, not 1200 as she was previously. This extra 700 cal per day will be so helpful in ensuring she can eat more food whilst dieting and thus lower stress on the body whilst doing so.

The other consideration for those who are not Susan, who we may assume are attempting a diet from a better place where they have not chronically undereaten, is to not diet too aggressively!

It is the biggest diet fail I see and is the most common source of failure for sustained fat loss.

People begin a new diet and immediately throw themselves on aggressive calorie deficits or follow the latest crash dieting fad.
A juice cleanse.
Ketogenic dieting.
Carnivore.
Paleo.

They cut all carbohydrates for an arbitrary amount of time.

These rapid attempts at gaining instant reward for their efforts unfortunately ultimately lead them to becoming unstuck.

They end up starving, foggy-headed, stressed, and anxious. These extreme diets often lead to long-lasting negative implications for lowering of testosterone in men, disruptions of ovulation for women, and massive disruptions in appetite regulation for the long term.

Many who have dieted harshly will have experienced first-hand that it can take months to get their ravenous appetite to calm down, for example, no matter how much food they eat!

This is our body trying to restore homeostasis.

Short-term aggressive drops in weight in caveman times likely meant starvation and this life-or-death scenario caused the body to make some very clever hormonal adaptations.

It would slow our BMR. It would increase insulin resistance to ensure any carbohydrates we do eat we can store as fat so we have energy stores to stave off this starvation!

It would increase cortisol output to liberate more stored energy in the face of less incoming food and it would up regulate fat storage to ensure any calories we do consume do get stored for later!

This is the evolutionary biology working against you when you crash diet.

This is the long-term biological baggage, that stopped us from starving to death in our ancestors' times, that is directly destroying your dieting success in modern times when you go on a 7-day juice cleanse!

SO HOW DO I DIET PROPERLY?

So, when dieting, follow the research of Dr. Bill Campbell.

Dr. Bill Campbell is a professor of Exercise Science and director of the Performance and Physique Enhancement Laboratory at the University of South Florida.

Bill has outlined two very simple rules for a successful fat loss phase that ensures it is sustainable.

Firstly, eat high protein. It is the body's catcher's mitt against dieting leading to unfavourable outcomes like loss of lean muscle mass as opposed to body fat. He recommends 1.6 g of protein per 1 kg of body weight in my interview with Bill on the *Wotsupp podcast*. So, a 100 kg male should consume 160 g protein to ensure maintenance of muscle mass, maintenance of a strong BMR, and better long-term body composition.

Secondly, he recommends not exceeding a 20% calorie deficit. This means if your maintenance calories are 3000 for example for the 100 kg male above, then 20% is 600 calories.

We also know that with weight loss, it is best to go slow and steady.

So, if 20% is the ceiling of where we can go in terms of a calorie deficit, it would be smart to start smaller at say a 10% calorie deficit to give us room to move when the weight loss starts slowing down.

This would mean this 100 kg male should be on a high protein diet of at least 160 g protein, and should not go below 2400 calories during this fat loss phase to ensure optimal and sustainable fat loss. Ideally, he would start at a 10% deficit, which would mean starting at 2700 calories for a period of time until weight loss stalls for more than 3 consecutive weeks (remember weight loss in not linear so weekly changes are way too rapid).

To calculate your maintenance (AKA TDEE) caloric requirement, there is a host of TDEE calculators available on the internet such as *www.tdeecalculator.net*, or you can start with a good ballpark by taking your body weight in pounds (weight in kg x 2.2) and multiplying it by 13–15.

So, for this active 100 kg male, his weight in pounds is

100 x 2.2 = 220 lbs.
220 x 13 = 2860
220 x 15 = 3300

The average is 3080 calories.

A 12-WEEK WORKED EXAMPLE
OF A DIETING PHASE

Dr. Bill Campbell's recommendation of no more than 20% when going into a calorie deficit would lead me to recommend starting at 10% as the initial calorie deficit.

Therefore, weeks 1–4, I would start with a 10% caloric deficit applied, that would look like starting at 2772 calories with at least 160 g of protein as your starting point.

Weeks 5–9, we would then drop calories to a 15% deficit of 2618 cal for a further 2–4-week period until weight loss is stalled again for several consecutive weeks.

Finally, for weeks 9–12 we could go to a 20% calorie deficit of 2464 cal to round out the final weeks of fat loss.

This would be a great starting point to start mapping out a 12-week dieting template for what is an appropriate calorie deficit for your fat loss phase that doesn't have your body swimming in a bath of cortisol!

1. Excessive Exercise and Overtraining

This source of stress, whilst common, applies to those who have athletic pursuits and who train regularly. If you are not someone who weight trains regularly or undergoes some kind of intense exercise on a weekly basis, you can skip over this stressor. But for those whom this does apply to, read on attentively because whilst training is a good stress on the body, it is still a stressor!

The premise of exercise is imposing a stressor onto your body with an attempt to gain a positive adaptation to this stress. In the weights room, we are applying stress to specific muscles, with 'progressive overload' being the goal of the weekend warrior! To subject our musculature to increasing load and volume over time is the name of the game!

But it is worth noting, whilst these are only small, incremental increases in weight or repetitions performed, nothing is truly easy for the body in this equation. That is the point after all, by applying greater work each time, we overload the muscle, causing a stressor that the body then rushes to repair using increases in muscle protein synthesis (MPS), modulating inflammation, and driving the parasympathetic nervous system to encourage rest and repair.

Where this falls apart, is when we are attempting to progressively overload in the weights room, whilst unknowingly, also progressively overloading stress in the world outside the gym at the same time!

Many trainees can empathise that a hard week in the gym can be a job in and of itself to recover from. By Friday, you have gone through 3–5 heavy sessions and the body is letting you know it. It is DOMS galore; you are sore and stiff and inflamed. The perfect environment in a normal environment to create signals in the body that these muscles need some R&R to start rebuilding ASAP!

However, what most of us do instead is spend the entire week redlining in our sympathetically driven, high stress lifestyles, and spend the majority of our waking time outside the gym in unknowing flight-or-fight mode.

As we covered in earlier chapters, the parasympathetic rest-and-digest nervous system is what is required to rebuild and repair our body, especially with regards to muscle tissue.

So, where overtraining comes in, it is not so much about the workout itself being way too much for the average person. It's more of a recoverability issue because we are spending near-zero time at rest-and-digest, and almost all of our time in the catabolic state that is flight-or-fight.

A catabolic state refers to a state where your body is breaking things down, using them either as fuel typically, which is the exact opposite of an anabolic state. An anabolic state is rebuilding and repairing and synthesise new tissue mode. Funnily enough, when we are in flight-or-fight we are in a catabolic state and when we are parasympathetic, we are in an anabolic state.

So, if our week is full of stressors with poor sleep quality, highly demanding jobs to attend to, kids to juggle, and only 5–6 hours of some pretty average sleep per night, then we are effectively constantly in this catabolic flight-or-fight state!

This makes recovery from exercise very difficult and something that does actually contribute to a state of 'overtraining'.

Overtraining can be defined as a state where the demands placed on the body outstrip the body's ability to recover. In the above example, if you have a boatload of life stressors to contend with, then it is very likely your ability to engage in parasympathetic repair work is very low, and thus overtraining will likely become a source of cortisol output for you very quickly.

For, progressive overload only works if you can recover from the stress we place on the muscle. Otherwise, it's just applying a stress for the hell of it, with no positive adaptations!

Because recovery is where the growth of muscle or burning of fat comes from. Not being in flight-or-fight 24/7.

So, this paints an interesting scenario that explains how exercise and overtraining is a common source of stress for the daily gym-goer:

1. High lifestyle stressors detract from your ability to recover from hard exercise.
2. Poor recovery over time leads to a state of overtraining where positive adaptations cease, leading to a state of overtraining.
3. Overtraining is a well-known state of high stress hormone output as the body recognises it cannot recover with the resources it has on hand with the demands placed upon it.
4. Increased stress hormone output from being overtrained contributes to bullet point 1 above, and so round and round we go on the Ferris wheel of cortisol!

It is a cyclical issue, and one that we can attack with a few simple steps, to reduce this common source of stress for many people who exercise regularly.

STEP ONE – ASSESS RECOVERABILITY BY LOOKING AT EXTERNAL STRESS OUTSIDE OF THE GYM FLOOR:

As we mentioned above, stress outside the gym will directly impact your recovery. You have to be in an anabolic state to recover stressed muscle tissue from hard exercise and this means you need to assess how much time you spend in rest-and-digest vs flight-or-fight throughout your week. If you are not sure how to assess this, start by tallying which of the sources of stress from this chapter apply to your daily life. Depending on how many sources of stress you have, this will indicate how much time you are likely in flight-or-fight vs rest-and-digest.

STEP TWO – MODIFY WORKLOAD IN THE GYM TO SUIT YOUR ACTUAL RECOVERABILITY

This is what has made the most personal difference to the author in recent times. Running a growing business with nearly a dozen staff, having parental commitments, and frequent inter-state travel meant my lifestyle stressors were sky-high!

I used to train five to even six times a week and wondered why I always had stubborn fat on my lower stomach, why my niggles from an old shoulder injury never settled down, and why I wasn't able to push past certain weights each week on squats or heavy compounds.

Essentially, my time in flight-or-fight was the vast majority of my time outside the gym, and my time in rest and digestion was near zero.

So, I decided to modify my training from 5–6 days per week to only 4 days. Now, this was actually hard to do. My younger years in bodybuilding and having a strong work ethic led to me believing fervently that if I wanted progress, I had to work harder than I currently am.

If I wanted more muscle and I was training five times, then the answer was to train six!

But I assessed my stress levels outside the gym, went with my science-based logic over my 'gym bro logic' and dropped training to 4 days a week.

Within the first week, my stomach started moving. It was mental!

I hadn't changed anything with food yet either.

I noticed my shoulder settled down completely by week 2, and I am happy to report, hasn't flared up much since.

I started progressing weekly in my recorded lifts, going up 5–10 kg per week on squats like clockwork.

So, what happened? How could training less means more results?

Well, quite simply, the stress on the body lowered when I went from 6 days to 4 per week. This meant the stress I was placing on my body started falling within my ability to recover and so the positive adaptations to exercise started creeping in nicely!

I knew the science and theory of why this would work but it was incredibly encouraging when I executed it for myself, and it paid off big time!

So in summary of step 2, I highly recommend you assess your lifestyle and stressors outside the gym before you throw your-self at your next 10x10 German volume training block.

If you have a high demand job, family at home, financial stresses, and a coffee addiction, then don't go expecting your body to be able to recover from being bashed 6 days a week in the gym!

Instead, acknowledge what life currently looks like for you, and modify your training volume to suit.

PRACTICAL VOLUME MODIFICATION:

If you are in a very high stress lifestyle, I would recommend stripping back total sessions to 4 days per week, with 4 exercises per session.

Start off with a simple 3 working sets per exercise, making for 4 gym sessions with 12 working sets in each session (48 total working sets for the week). This is a good base point many should be able to recover from, in my anecdotal experience.

If you are in the low stress category, then you can likely ratchet that volume up to say 5 sessions a week doing 4–5 exercises and 3 working sets each session. Making total volume 5 sessions/week with 12–15 working sets per session per week (60–75 working sets per week).

Knowing the high and low end of volume, now you can modify your current training with these anecdotal recommendations on volume in mind!

STEP THREE – ENSURE CALORIC INTAKE/NUTRITION IS ADEQUATE TO SUPPORT YOUR EXERCISE GOALS

There is a whole section on undereating above that covers the solid principles on how to have nutrition that is appropriate if fat loss is your goal.

So, not having to dwell on a fat loss focus, we can cast our attention to the other end of the spectrum of muscle growth.

So, to ensure you are aiming for muscle growth and want your nutrition to support that, use the equation found in the 'Undereating' chapter to calculate your TDEE (maintenance calories). This is simply body weight in pounds x 13–15 and taking the average of the two numbers as your starting point.

For muscle growth, we then add a small 10% surplus to ensure our body has adequate resources with which to grow muscle tissue.

Protein should be 1.6 g of protein per kilogram of body weight.

The rest should be made up of plenty of carbohydrates (which are protective against cortisol, thanks to our old friend insulin) and healthy fats.

Using the example of a 100 kg male with a maintenance of 3000 calories, this would mean eating 3300 calories to support muscle growth.

This calorie surplus will minimise stress on the body by ensuring there are plenty of resources to spare to build that muscle tissue you are chasing!

Most people undereat without knowing it, as we have covered above. So, by ensuring you follow the guidelines in the 'Undereating' chapter and the guidance for a calorie surplus set out there, you know you won't be overtraining due to your nutrition letting you down!

STEP 4 – ADD IN SUPPLEMENTATION TO DRIVE RECOVERY IF BUDGET ALLOWS

There are three supplements I would recommend for recovery.

Protein powders to ensure the 1.6 g of protein/kg body weight is being hit

Essential amino acids or BCAAs (both are effective but EAAs are preferred)

Adrenal and sleep supplements (will be covered in extensive depth later under the chapter 'Supplement Hacks to Make You Bulletproof', so we won't go into depth here)

BRANCHED CHAIN AMINO ACIDS (BCAAS)

These were traditionally the heavy lifters of almost every intra workout formula. BCAAs were the first combination of amino acids popularised as a recovery aid, endurance potentiator, as well as helping preserve lean muscle mass when dieting and training intensely.

BCAAs have since been superseded by the more comprehensive 9 essential amino acids as the main start of modern intra workout formulas. However, it is worthy of note that BCAAs are part of the 9 EAA group. So, in the argument of what is best, BCAA or EAA, interestingly EAAs ARE BCAAs, plus 6 additional amino acids that more comprehensively stimulate muscle protein synthesis and aid performance.

So, let's have a look at BCAAs, what they are made up of, and when to use them!

WHAT ARE THEY?

BCAAs refers to a Branched Chain configuration of the amino acids:

- Leucine
- Iso-Leucine
- Valine

These are three of the most anabolic amino acids in a protein polypeptide chain, with leucine being a particularly anabolic amino acid that is doing the bulk of the work in activating MTOR pathways to stimulate protein synthesis and repair.

HOW DO THEY WORK?

In simple terms, the role of BCAAs are centred around recovery, primarily by preventing muscle break down and in so doing, making physically recovering from a workout a far quicker process. The less a muscle is broken down, the less it has to be repaired before new growth can occur. Additionally, by stimulating muscle protein synthesis, leucine minimises the catabolic effects of intense training.

BCAAs also have the unique ability to be utilised as an incredibly fast burning fuel source, if glycogen stores and available glucose has been otherwise depleted. To this end, if your nutritional needs are not being met, if you are in a calorie deficit, or if you are not consuming adequate carbohydrates around training times, then using BCAAs during training will prevent your body from breaking down muscle tissue, via the process of gluconeogenesis to create glucose to fuel exercise and the Kreb Cycle. So, having BCAAs present to be utilised as a fuel source will act secondarily to spare muscle tissue during the catabolic period during training.

TIPS TO KNOW

BCAAs are most commonly found in a 2:1:1 ratio in nature, and in almost all studies, a 2:1:1 ratio has shown the highest assimilation and utilisation by muscle in terms of muscle protein synthesis, etc.

DOSAGE

5–10 grams is ideal as the best dosage of 2:1:1 BCAAs for increasing MTOR and thus, protein synthesis, although studies have shown as little as 5.6 g to be effective.

ESSENTIAL AMINO ACIDS (EAAS)

Recent research has shown that superior results are seen in elevating muscle protein synthesis, when BCAAs are accompanied by the other six essential amino acids. It seems that more complete the amino acids profile of the supplement, the greater the muscle protein response remains elevated.

EAAs are seen to be the preferred choice to BCAAs alone, in recent formulations we see hitting the Australian marketplace.

WHAT ARE THEY?

These essential amino acids are called essential because these are the amino acids that your body must source from diet or supplementations, because we cannot make them ourselves.

This means you MUST supplement with them, as your body cannot directly create them as it can with the non-essential amino acids.

Funnily enough, the nine Essential Amino Acids include the three BCAAs as well. So, EAAS are BCAAs as well as six more amino acids.

HOW DO THEY WORK?

Interestingly, BCAAs alone will elevate muscle protein synthesis (MPS) for 1–2 hours post ingestion. After this point, it will return to baseline, which is not the case with EAAS which have a more complete amino acid profile.

This is because the amino acid profile is incomplete and after the leucine is metabolised to elevate MPS, unless all amino acids are present to facilitate the rest of the tasks a complete protein does in the body, it will return to baseline.

Therefore, for longer bouts of exercise over 90 mins, and for a complete amino acid supplement that can be utilised between meals as a standalone replacement to dietary protein, a supplement containing both BCAAs and EAAs is ideal for keeping MPS levels elevated and minimise catabolism/kick-start repair processes.

WHAT ARE THE 9 EAAS?

- Leucine
- Isoleucine
- Valine
- Threonine
- Histidine
- Methionine
- Tryptophan
- Phenylalanine
- Lysine

DOSAGE:

Studies show a dose as low as 6 grams of EAAs will significantly increase MPS. Ideally, the author recommends 10 grams, however, for solid weight training.

PROTEIN POWDERS

Whether they are plant-based (pea or rice proteins), or whey-based (whey protein isolates, whey protein concentrates, casein), or collagen-based protein powders have similar characteristics.

They will increase MPS (muscle protein synthesis), making them an excellent tool to help recovery from exercise.

They also contain on average 20–30 g of protein per scoop, the equivalent of 150 g of lean meat, approximately. This makes them an excellent alternative to having to eat mountains of chicken breast to hit your protein targets that will, in turn, facility muscle growth and recovery from exercise.

The best timing for protein shakes is pre- or post-workout, or at any other meal in the day that is a bit light on protein and needs a decent bump to get the protein goals up!

ADRENAL SUPPLEMENTS

These are a blessed supplemental category.

Adrenal supplements refer to the family of supplements designed to help improve our response to stress, that lowers our cortisol levels, and that can improve our resilience to stress.

They often feature adaptogens, which are a family of herbs that help our bodies adapt to the stressors imposed upon them by our crazy modern lifestyles.

Adaptogenic herbs that help to lower stress and foster resilience in our nervous system include:

- Ashwagandha (300 mg twice per day)
- Rhodiola (250–400 mg)
- Schisandra (250–400 mg)
- Panax or Siberian Ginseng (250–1000 mg)
- Lemon Balm (300–1000 mg)
- Holy Basil (a.k.a. Tulsi) (500–1000 mg)

All of these herbs have similar properties, in that they modulate the HPA axis to either secrete less cortisol in the event of something stressful happening, or alternatively, they assist in helping lower cortisol at key times such as in the evenings. They also typically help lower perceived stress or anxiety throughout the day and assist greatly with sleep quality and general restlessness.

Other supplements that aren't necessarily adaptogens but that assist people under high stress, and therefore, come under the adrenally beneficial banner include:

- GABA (500–1500 mg)
- L-Theanine (100–200 mg)
- Taurine (1000–5000 mg)
- Glycine (1000–5000 mg split into 2–3 doses)
- Passionflower Extract (250–1000 mg taken before bed)
- Valerian Root (250–750 mg taken before bed)
- Magnesium (200–400 mg of elemental yield Magnesium)

These supplements help in various ways to module GABA. When stress levels are chronically elevated, we tend to see that the GABA levels in our brain are low. GABA is an inhibitory neurotransmitter that is responsible for calming of our minds. It is often highest before bed and promotes sensations of calmness, well-being, and improves sleep latency.

Many of these supplements are amazing at either increasing GABA activity in the brain to counteract the negative effects of chronic stress. They will contribute to sleep quality, calming of a busy, stressed mind, and will definitely lower perceived anxiety and stress during the day when used at the right dosages.

The dosages listed are what I have had good success formulating with, to help reduce stress and anxiety, improve sleep, and recover from chronic stress. They are what I have found to be effective and are backed by thousands of customers using my formulations from anecdotal data as well as countless studies.

The data is quite amazing at showing how strongly these herbs can modulate cortisol. For example, ashwagandha was shown to lower cortisol by 32% when taken twice per day at 300 mg for 6 weeks.

A 32% reduction in cortisol is massive!

There is amazing data showing how lemon balm and holy basil reduced perceived stress and had an 85% remission from insomnia symptoms (i.e., 85% of subjects with stress-induced insomnia slept well after supplementation with holy basil).

The ginseng family has been used for centuries in herbal medicine to increase resilience, endurance, vitality, strength of immune systems, and become bulletproof to stress!

Adrenal supplements should be one of your first lines of defence when tackling a stressful lifestyle head-on!

- **Uncertainty and Large Life Changes** – This category falls more under the psychosocial causes of stress for the body. We cover the cost of emotional stress on cortisol later in the book, in Part 2, but for now, to summarise, we can simply look at the world's uncertainty and change.

Our body hates both these things and has dozens of biological features designed to counter these two elements of life.

In fact, our body thrives best when it is certain, safe, and our day looks predictable. Homeostasis occurs with the least effort when the environment is steady, predictable, and reliable.

So, it is no wonder that uncertainty or large life changes would cause significant angst and mental chatter, leading to increased cortisol.

- **Blood Sugar Fluctuations** – Whenever our blood sugar drops below an optimal range, our body releases cortisol to activate glucagon and liberate stored fuel and dump it into our bloodstream. This process is covered extensively in the 'Nutrition' chapters of this book in Part 2.

So, to keep it brief, as we described above, every time you have fluctuations in blood sugar then your body will secrete cortisol to liberate stored blood sugar. Therefore, blood sugar fluctuations are common sources of stress for the body.

Now blood sugar may be fluctuating due to:

- Infrequent meal timings
- Intermittent fasting and other fasting practices
- Having caffeine on an empty stomach, particularly, before breakfast
- Stress
- Insulin resistance and high body fat levels

So, what should we do?

We need to keep blood sugar stable as much as possible. This can be achieved by eating adequate carbohydrates in the first place. If we take in adequate fuel then we shouldn't be as likely to have to dip into our stores via cortisol. Furthermore, these carbohydrates should be ideally accompanied by a protein and/ or a modest fat source. Fats serve to slow the release of blood sugar and make our insulin releases far more modest.

They should also be from whole food and low glycaemic sources during the day if we are not physically active.

If you are in a desk job, we can't have you slamming bags of gummy bears in the name of stress reduction! You will end up pre-diabetic before ever being chill enough to justify the work-out on your pancreas!

Think complex carbs like wholemeal breads, grains, sour-doughs, sweet potatoes, pumpkins, white potatoes, oats, and fibrous vegetables.

Now for active people who resistance train, this may also mean consuming a nice carbohydrate-rich meal before and after exercise as well, to ensure adequate fuelling for the training and lowering cortisol in the hours after your workout.

For most people, fuelling adequately for a 60-minute workout would look like 30–60 g of carbohydrates that are medium to high GI an hour, before your workout and again after your workout.

Think bananas, honey, white bread, white rice, and fast digesting carbohydrates like cereals.

Whether you are athletic or not, we also want to ensure that our insulin sensitivity is nice and high, so that our body doesn't over secrete insulin when eating carbohydrate-rich meals.

Insulin resistance is a major cause of blood sugar fluctuations and therefore, cortisol spikes. We cover this in much more depth in Part 2 of this book where we analyse the relationship between cortisol and insulin. But to improve insulin sensitivity, we want to be physically active and also keep our body fat levels nice and low (10–20% for men and 20–30% for women). We also want to minimise inflammation and stress as both massively drive insulin resistance. We also want to optimise sleep quality. Following one poor night's sleep, we increase our insulin resistance by 31% according to the Muscle Expert podcast host Ben Pakulski, previous professional bodybuilder and now author.

So, now here you have some action items above and we also want to look at one last thing, which is timing.

To summarise these action items, eating regular, lower glycaemic carbohydrate meals throughout the day, and exercise will help keep a steady supply of glucose in the blood and therefore remove the need for cortisol to liberate any stored glycogen.

Furthermore, our carbohydrates would ideally be consumed alongside a protein and would be from whole food sources.

We also need to manage stress and optimise sleep quality. Finally, don't slam your morning coffee on an empty stomach before breakfast! This is when cortisol is already at its peak and having a stimulant on an empty stomach would send it skyrocketing.

That excessive cortisol will get all the fuel it can, dumped into the bloodstream causing significant fluctuations in blood sugar before you even have your first meal!

PART 2

**TURNING THE TIDE ON
CHRONIC STRESS – A LIFE
RAFT FOR THOSE SWIMMING
IN AN OCEAN OF CORTISOL**

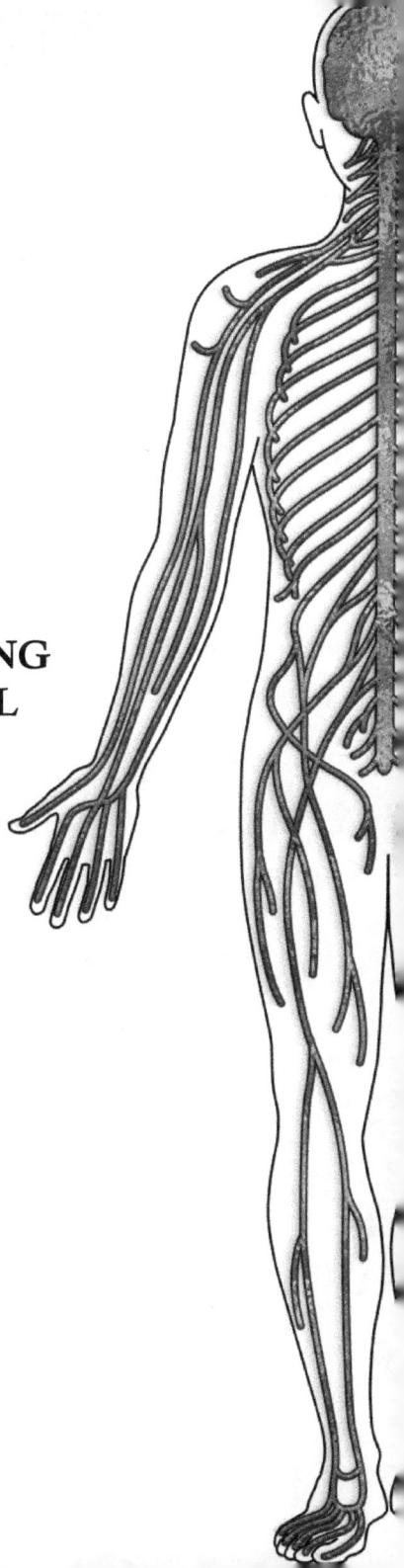

Part 2 of this book is all about switching gears.

Part 1 of the book so far has been all about the doom and gloom!

We outlined every single issue with stress as it plays out on your nervous system.

We looked at how it impacts us negatively, how we looked at common sources of stress, and how it plays out when it is chronically elevated.

But to stop there, would not be carrying out the mission statement of this book!

The purpose of authoring this text was to give you, the reader, all the tools you need to help make you bulletproof to this crazy burden we all face on a daily basis and make your nervous system into an unbeatable force!

Part 2 of the book is where we do just this!

This part of the book is now all about the psychological and physical rituals and practices we can implement into our daily lives to help make us bulletproof to stress!

I have endeavoured to make this section as comprehensive as possible and have done so by planning a thorough assault on cortisol management for you reading along at home.

This comprehensive assault starts with the psychological approach to stress management and how we can shift our perspectives and exercise a little bit of relativity to help frame better, what we interpret as stressful in the first place.

We cover a lot in this section, also on how repressed and unresolved emotional trauma can be a major stressor and how unpacking this can be an excellent tool in removing a silent killer of many, in terms of chronic stress exposure.

Next up, we deep dive into some daily practises that, when adopted, can help to give a means of maintaining the clear and conscious headspace required to fight the good fight!

By this, I mean that to be able to do much of the psychological work required to process and release repressed emotional baggage, or practise relativity and higher-order thinking, one must maintain a clear and level headspace.

Doing the daily practices I will suggest, will greatly aid in maintaining such a headspace.

From the mental health focus, we will then shift gears into the more physical practices we can use to make us resilient to stress.

We will look at the positive impacts of different types of exercise, ice baths, some nutritional strategies, and breathwork!

By the end of Part 2 of this book, you will have a whole arsenal of practises to improve your physical and mental health to tackle stress and make your nervous system bulletproof!

THE PSYCHOLOGY OF STRESS MANAGEMENT AND NERVOUS SYSTEM REGULATION

The more I researched on all areas of the body and its complex systems, the more I realised that the most positive results are always achieved by the most comprehensive approaches.

This is also true for regulation of the nervous system, and so to apply this comprehensive solution to the management of stress and indeed becoming bulletproof, one major area I personally overlooked for a very long time was the management of the psychological contributing factors to stress on the body.

For the author, this path of discovery of the impacts of emotions and trauma and all of its complexities has been a mixed journey, but one that has led to a place of clarity that I wanted to share with you, the reader.

The first discovery, as I touched on in Chapter 1, was that the body doesn't know the difference between an emotional stress vs a physical stress.

It is an identical stress response whether you just lost a leg in a horrific accident or are getting divorced.

The emotional stress response holds no difference in the body to that of the physical.

So, knowing this, we demonstrated in earlier chapters, that to tackle stress in the body we cannot neglect the psychology!

Repressed or unprocessed emotions are indeed a very potent source of chronically elevated stress hormones in the body.

IMPACT OF REPRESSED EMOTION AND TRAUMA ON STRESS HORMONES AND HEALTH

Gabor Mate is a Canadian physician and psychology buff who specialises in the impacts of trauma, emotional regulation, and repressed emotions' health impacts on the body.

This was explored in depth in his International best-selling book *When the Body Says No, The Cost of Hidden Stress.* In this book, Gabor explores the cases of dozens of patients he saw in a clinical setting with autoimmune diseases and cancers, and began to psychoanalyse them. He explores that there is a link between repressed emotion and trauma with chronically elevated stress in the body, which he theorises leads to health conditions and illnesses.

The idea that the body treats repressed emotional baggage as a source of long-term stress was demonstrated in the book, by Gabor interviewing multiple patients about their lives before their serious illnesses, and asking them questions pertaining to their childhoods, relationships, and lives.

Many of the patients started sharing some very common grounds that became the underpinning thesis of his work in the book. And that was, that they all had repression of emotion, an inability to express healthy anger, and had repressed trauma that had not been addressed.

These patients were all seemingly saintly individuals.

They were the carers of sick children.

Loving wives, who would look after their families, often engaging in extracurricular school activities, running themselves ragged to ensure their children had the best childhoods.

Putting everyone and everything before themselves.

They were public servants and even doctors themselves in some cases, who continued to help others until the day they passed.

They were the people pleasers, those who struggled to say no.

Those who could give endlessly to others but when they were faced with their own issues, struggled to give themselves the time of the day to care for their own health concerns.

In fact, when many became sick they were more worried about how those around them would be affected by the news, than they were themselves.

These people all had these common traits – an almost inability to prioritise the self.

They were unable to face the hard facts that they were in perilous health and often distracted themselves by returning straight to work, or in some cases, even trying to continue caring for their loved ones despite being on death row themselves.

Simply put, in harrowing circumstances, they couldn't express themselves and what they were feeling, and in almost all cases, ignored their health concerns and actively made themselves busier, which is a very common practise of avoidance for the types of people Gabor studies.

Now the link that was drawn was that these chronic illnesses, such as cancers and autoimmune issues were due to these patients' inability to have healthy anger, or to turn their attention inward and address their own emotions in hard situations, but rather practising avoidance and engaging in distracting work in their lives.

Gabor theorises that the inability of his avoidant, people pleasing, self-sacrificing patients, to explore their own feelings and processing of emotions over their lifespan, led to chronic elevations of stress hormone physiology playing out.

That is, the chronic repression of emotion and pent-up psychological load led to chronic elevations in cortisol, thereby affecting immune system function and over time, their health.

Some powerful findings he had in his book were that those who experienced stress during isolation, with no significant other to share and process their emotions with, were nine times more likely to develop breast cancer, for example!

Or that parents who were carers of sick children were four times more likely to have cardiac-related fatalities, such as heart attacks or strokes.

So, with these harrowing statistics coming to light through studies from prestigious universities, it became obvious that one big foundational step to 'becoming bulletproof' to stress is addressing repressed emotions and processing (emotionally speaking) our stressful situations, if and when they arise, not holding to these feelings for weeks or months or years!

So how do we best do this?

How do we process and express emotions to stop them from becoming a contributing stressor to our lives, rather than an opportunity to reduce stress and anxiety?

Well, this must be a two-pronged approach.

Firstly, we must process the stored trauma the body carries already.

It is clear from Gabor's work that the stored and repressed emotions and trauma, are health-threatening sources of stress, so, we must start by first removing the source of stress in the first place.

Then secondly, we can also borrow from the philosophy of several schools, in how we frame our current lives to better relativise if a situation is stressful to begin with!

After all, through controlling our perspectives of a given situation comes the ability to decide if a situation is stressful or not in the first place. And this may well be our best shot at avoiding the need for a stress response from the body, at all!

Perspective is the lens we view the world with, and so, by learning to better give context to life events, we can start to shape how our nervous system perceives and thus responds to stressors.

We can stop the stress response before it even begins!

STEP ONE – PROCESSING EMOTIONS AND TRAUMA

Now self admittedly, this topic is well and truly out of my wheelhouse at the time of writing this book. I have spent a decade studying the chemistry and tangible physical responses to stress, hormones, and physiology. Never had I looked at the implications of emotions in the body.

And I think, it is very important that authors confess their limitations so as to ensure the utmost academic integrity is maintained and the audience understands the potential limitations of a body of work by an author, from these reflections.

However, through the recent undertaking of a personal journey of self-awareness, inner child work, ravenous consumption of content looking at childhood conditioning and healing trauma, doing breathwork, journaling, and extensive mindfulness work, I have garnered a slightly above-average ability to point you in the right direction of some greater minds than my own on this topic, and have come up with a bit of a personally recommended approach to processing and dealing with previous trauma or emotion.

Therefore, this section of the book is more a summary of my opinion on the works of some of the authors I have enjoyed, and a distilled personal viewpoint based on this reading, as to what may help you start your emotional and trauma processing journey.

Some of these authors that have influenced my personal views on this topic include many of the greats, such as Eckhart Tolle, Friedrich Nietzsche, Carl Jung, Gabor Mate, and Brene Brown.

I have also enjoyed and been influenced by the more contemporary works, in parts by Chris Cheers, Michael Bunting, Carl Lemieux, and Roxie Nafousi.

So, now that the appropriate acknowledgements and limitations have been made, where to begin?

From what I could gather from the consumption of content on this topic, the early steps to releasing or processing emotions were to first 'look under the hood' so to speak, at what might be stored or repressed in you now. How can we process what we aren't aware of after all?

For me, this started by looking at childhood.

The reason I started there was that many of the underpinning theories around modern psychology are based on the works of the greats, like Carl Jung, Nietzsche, and Freud who postulated that childhood was where much of our emotional blueprints that set us up for emotional well-being or trauma occur.

For the uninitiated like myself, this also appealed as a place to start because I (like many I am sure) had no idea where to start!

So, what better place than the beginning?

It almost guarantees that by starting at the literal start, you in the very worst-case scenario, won't have missed anything in your timeline!

Even if you were blessed with a textbook-perfect childhood, you have at least done your emotional diligence in taking stock of your entire timeline, rightly so, starting where you should, at the start!

Going back to childhood and looking at how we interacted with our care giving figures during these formative years, would fall under the broad umbrella of 'inner child work' and gives an excellent indicator of where to start, and what may be the earliest sources of our stored trauma.

It also will inform us about how we 'attach' as adults, that is, how we form relationships with significant others in our lives.

This is termed attachment theory, and is another excellent area to further study if relationship breakdowns or struggles have been a source of stress for you as an adult.

British psychologist John Bowlby was the first attachment theorist.

He described attachment in his book *Attachment and Loss* as a 'lasting psychological connectedness between human beings'.

Bowlby was interested in understanding the anxiety and distress that children experience when separated from their primary caregivers.

These distresses that come from the dynamic between you as an infant and your caregiver are exactly what a host of modern psychologists agree, is a common source of long-forgotten repressed trauma.

This makes an excellent starting point to unpacking your personal repressed emotional baggage, and thus beginning your journey towards processing (and thus releasing) this source of chronic stress on the body to ultimately make us bulletproof to stress!

To shed some light on how this may look practically, I will share how looking at inner child work and attachment theory helped me personally unpack and process a lot of trauma that was a massive source of stress for me. Crazy part is, I didn't even know it was a source of stress for me, it was all buried so deep in the subconscious!

So, to give this personalised practical look at how you too may start undertaking this work, I will summarise how I tackled my own 'work'. The first thing I was instructed to do was look at some patterns of behaviour as an adult that no longer served me, or that were directly causing issues in my current life.

For me, being a workaholic was definitely one.

In relation to romantic life as well, much of my sources of stress had also been relationship breakdowns, so, this was another area I tackled as part of my priority list.

Starting with the workaholic patterning, this was a massive source of stress for me.

I simply didn't have a second gear.

My work ethic was so strong that my body would break before my mind did.

I had an inability to work at any other pace or capacity other than at one that led to frequent burn outs, relationship issues, and even physical health deterioration.

It was a flat stick, all the time, for decades!

Even during university, I had three jobs. I had my first job at 12, working after school in year 7 at high school.

I had a second job I took during school holidays as well, so by the time I left high school in 2008, I had already been working for 5 years.

Now, the hard part is that this immense work ethic was rewarded by society and was very productive for building a successful business.

It accelerated me in any occupation I had, any employer who hired me was thrilled, and when I started my business, working like a maniac paid dividends!

But it was still very clear that it was causing major problems for me emotionally, relationally, socially, and was something I identified as a source of chronic stress for my body.

So, my work in trying to remove this as a source of chronic stress was unpacking why I struggled to switch off.

Why couldn't I just work at a normal pace?

Why couldn't I be content when I was burnt out and needed to take a day off?

Why did I feel the need to work all the time and feel guilty taking a day off?

Starting with the early childhood work, I realised that it had origins in my upbringing.

Coming from a working-class, blue-collar family growing up on a farm, work ethic was drummed into me from an early age. It was something my parents passed on as one of their top priorities and ensured I valued it too!

I also recognised (through guided work with a therapist) that work ethic was also one of the few things I received praise for as a young person. It was always praised and was on a very short list of things that got praise for me as a young boy.

So, the pattern started to reveal itself.

Work ethic was reinforced as a priority by caregivers. I was then given positive reinforcement in the form of encouragement and praise when I did work hard as a young man.

All the whilst, almost nothing else I did received praise.

So it is easy to see from the works of psychologists and philosophers like Jung and Bowlby that if a child is told something is good, and then praised exclusively when doing that task, it will be learned very quickly by that child to continue that behaviour as it will be rewarded and given positive reinforcement.

It will also get that child's affection and what they interpret as attachment to their caregivers, making it almost a guarantee that that child will ongoingly continue to repeat that behaviour to get what all children need the most, love and attachment from their caregivers.

Now, by the time I was an adult, this was all firmly rooted in my subconscious. I didn't actively recall or reflect ever on my parents' conditioning towards work ethic, and it took direct conscious effort and reflection to recall it at all.

It was like an old record, playing in the background on repeat, blasting in the deafness of my subconscious:

Work = praise, and praise = love.

So, as an adult I carried out this subconscious patterning, and as an adult and in full control of my own life now, it's logical now looking back why I took it to the extreme.

The inner child craves that attachment desperately and so keeps subconsciously playing out the pattern of working hard, hoping the work ethic will get the praise and love shown as a child.

And as an adult, with no one to tell you otherwise or keep it in check, I kept playing this learned behavioural pattern out to an absurd extent.

All the whilst, oblivious to why I couldn't stop!

So, here is a perfect example of a source of stress that can come from deeply rooted, lifelong patterns of behaviour that are a direct result of some dysfunctional psychological adaptations.

When I started to realise this, it was a life-changing light bulb moment.

When I could see my own subconscious record player, playing on repeat, driving my dysfunctional behavioural patterning as an adult, it was as if I could see for the first time.

I had brought the subconscious into the light.

I had dragged up long-repressed emotions with these reflections that I had no idea were still stored in my body somewhere deeply.

It began flooding to the surface, recollections of not feeling adequate, or being praised or validated as a young boy unless it was directly due to showing some display of work ethic.

Remembering the lack of feeling of attachment and affection or positive reinforcement outside of these rare moments of praise.

All of this was coming back to me. But I had to look extremely hard, straining to see it at first. It was like trying to look through a foggy mirror, I could just start to make things out, but had to focus on everything I had, to bring these things into sharp focus.

It was amazing the emotions that came over in the following weeks and months of unpacking these early memories. Looking for the lack in my youth.

Looking for, when as a child I didn't feel loved or validated, or when my emotions weren't validated by parent figures.

I can see how we have no clue this is all going on in the background. All of us do to some extent. Ironically as well, childhood was seemingly a beautiful experience from my recollections, yet had so much unprocessed associated baggage and emotion tied to it.

I can't help but imagine what it must be like for someone carrying around the weight of the emotional baggage that would accrue, if they had actually had a hard upbringing as well, like many of us do?

What if one had grown up in poverty?

Or been physically or sexually abused?

Or had caregivers withhold love or be manipulative due to their own intergenerational trauma?

It is plain to see why so many people have subconsciously repressed emotional baggage contributing to their chronically elevated stresses.

Why the people in Gabor Mate's book ended up in the hospital bed, from unknowingly carrying around these huge emotional weights their whole lives without even knowing it?

For me, it was so liberating to start reflecting that many other patterns of behaviour I had as an adult were the result of these same conditioning patterns from my formative years. And so, one by one, I sought them out, reflected on them, and looked back into the early years, searching for the reason, why I am how I am!

It was so freeing, as I started working through these emotions that would come up as well, sometimes by talking about them with my therapist, or friends.

Other times, simply by acknowledging that I was feeling a given emotion, and letting it stay with me until it passed. Feeling into it, and letting it go, like a cloud drifting by, the emotions would eventually drift on after they had been acknowledged and felt.

And to me, in my personal and entirely unqualified opinion, this is how we process repressed emotional baggage (and in so doing start taking the chronic stress burden off our bodies). Or at least it was how I felt I did that for myself.

By first going deeper, scanning our subconscious, our early years, and the deepest corners of our beings. Looking for long-forgotten lessons from our younger selves.

Then, letting the associated memories, emotions, and feelings float up to the surface with them, and feeling them deeply and sincerely for as long as these feelings wish to stay.

For me, this was sometimes very intense.

Powerful waves of anger, or sadness, or whatever else had been lurking deep under there came to the surface.

I was incapable of functioning at times.

But as I went deeper and deeper and sat into that state, letting myself feel angry, or sad, or melancholy, the quicker they began retreating.

The emotions had done what they had craved to do all along.

Be brought into the light, been validated and experienced, and then allowed to move on.

Like ghosts that were trapped and couldn't pass to the other side, so too were stored emotions unable to leave the body until they had been properly processed.

Ironically too, once the patterns of behaviour like my workahol-ism were seen for what they truly were (a dysfunctional attempt of a child trying to get love from their parents), it became instantly simplified, how to drop the habitual overworking.

Once I recognised that my obsessive workaholic tendencies, that had ravaged many of my romantic and social relationships as an adult, were just a broken record playing out, being orchestrated by my inner child seeking love, it all dissolved in front of me.

The need to work dissipated.

The intensity with which I had thrown myself at work could ease. I started taking days off and not feeling guilty.

I started being compassionate towards myself.

I started giving myself time off and taking holidays, something I hadn't done in living memory!

Amazingly, with this came a huge physical transformation too. I dropped 5 kg out of nowhere on the scales, with my stomach disappearing with seemingly no other changes to diet or lifestyle.

I felt lighter.

I didn't feel so 'old' with regards to my inner dialogue and how I spoke to myself about life.

I am convinced now, that I had liberated such a huge source of stress for my body in starting to process some of these stored emotions, that I was experiencing the positive side effects of my nervous system regenerating.

I could almost feel the cortisol melting away, my perceived stress was so much lower too with day-to-day life.

I began seeking out the company of friends and colleagues and brought balance into my life, for the first time that I could recall. All of this was powerfully transformative, and I am thoroughly convinced would be for you too, reading along at home.

If you could take the time and face the dark of your own past, a very significant source of chronic stress could be washed away at its source!

You too could feel your nervous system finally be able to rest and could finally take some of the weights off your shoulders, that have been pulling you down subconsciously for a lifetime!

And what a noble quest that would be?

Knowing of self is ironically the final frontier for many of us as adults, which we typically don't come to until much later in life. But in this self-knowing comes the most profound benefits of all, and pursuit of this deep self-knowing cannot be stressed enough as a worthy crusade to embark upon!

PART TWO – SHIFTING PERSPECTIVE
TO FOSTER RESILIENCE TO STRESS:

As the title of this book implies, building resilience to stress is the goal of this text.

Stress is an unavoidable facet of modern living, but it is also less often discussed as the gateway to growth!

Stress is necessary to stimulate and challenge the body to produce an adaptation. Adaptations can be positive or negative depending on how resilient we become, and so, it is in our best interest to become bulletproof to the stressors life throws at us, so as to stack the deck in our favour and drive positive adaptations, versus the negative ones we experience when we are not resilient to stress.

So how can we shift how we engage with stress to rig the hand we are dealt, into driving positive adaptations vs just running us into the ground?

Perspective, my friends.

Perspective.

The lens with which we view the world is everything.

The way we engage with the world tells our nervous system a lot about whether it needs to be in 'flight-or-fight' vs 'rest-and-digest'.

As we covered in earlier chapters, our nervous system is constantly scanning our environment (4 times per second, in fact) looking for answers to the questions:

Am I safe?
Do I have shelter?

Do I have enough food?
Am I in a secure and predictable environment?

Our perception of the environment, therefore, modulates how we answer these questions. Take a contemporary example of an ice bath. The cold plunge has been popularised in recent years as a way to challenge your nervous system into some positive adaptations, challenge mental toughness, and overall just give an opportunity to do something bloody hard!

Now, let's examine how perspective can shape our nervous system's response to stressors. Let us use this example; if you take a fixed event, say a 3-minute cold plunge in 4 degrees icy cold water, and look at that experience with two separate people, both with different perspectives.

Person 1 climbs in, perceiving the ice bath as a positive event that will help boost their metabolism, lower inflammation, and give them an amazing feeling afterwards. They see it as a great opportunity to practise mindfulness and intentionally control their breathing during a hard event, eventually sinking into a nice deep breath cycle mid plunge. They emerge after their 3 minutes and really sit with the greatness of how alive they feel when they hop out, how proud they are they accomplished something hard, and they go on to tackle the day with an optimism nigh seen before!

The second person climbs in adopting the perspective, this experience will be brutal. They dread walking up to the side of the bath, contemplating how cold the ice will feel when they climb in. When they get in their breathing is jagged, with the only conscious thought being how long they need to endure this icy torture until they can get out, counting down the seconds! Tensing their shoulders, clenching their jaw, and breathing like they are in a 100 m sprint! They climb out, feel the burning of their skin and the coldness of the air on their goosebumps-ridden skin. They have just dragged themselves through hell!

Now, here is a perfect example of how two separate people can have an identical experience in a controlled environment matched to temperature and time, and through perception alone could have wildly different stress responses.

To the readers playing along at home with this worked example, do you want to take a punt on how this plays out for the two people in terms of perceptions and stress responses to this experience?

Well, it will play out a little something like this.

Person 1, who perceived the ice bath as a positive opportunity for growth and health improvements, will have a nervous system that will be mildly confronted, will recognise the positive intention set before getting in, and have a modest stress response that drives the positive adaptations ice baths are famous for.

Person 2, who just survived their own worst nightmare will have sky-high cortisol, with a stress response fitting to the perceived hell they have just survived! They will likely take a beating from the event, both in terms of their hormonal stress response and mentally, and likely carry around an ongoing stressful association with all future hard tasks to boot.

Same experience.

Two different perspectives.

Two entirely different stress responses.

It is now easy to apply this same logic to our daily lives.

It is clear now how perceptions are actually the master modulator of our nervous system, and thus, stress responses in our daily lives.

After all, if you lined up Persons 1 and 2 from the above example, and followed along their lives, even with identical experiences, living in the same town or working the same job, their perception of how stressful that life would be, would clearly be leagues apart.

The optimistic Person 1 vs the real soldier in Person 2, will, through perception alone, interpret life's trials and tribulations entirely differently. And in so doing, completely change the stress responses to life's hurdles in the process. Person 2 will be a train wreck, likely suffering from broken sleep, poor libido, low motivation, anxiety, and view every peak as insurmountable. Person 1 will see every trial as an opportunity for growth and positive adaptations, with modest stress responses to follow!

Person 2 will see every difficulty as a stressful, unjust, gruelling task and will guaranteed have a cortisol response to match!

Person 1 will go out into the world and thrive!

Perception is truly the king of our environment!

PERSPECTIVES TO ADOPT TO LESSEN THE BLOW OF STRESSFUL TIMES – A LESSON FROM THE STOICS

The Stoic philosophy can be an excellent perspective to adopt if looking to navigate uncertain and tough times without having to swim through an ocean of cortisol.

This concept is explored a lot in Brigid Delaney's book *Reasons Not to Worry-How to Be Stoic in Chaotic Times*. Delaney unpacks many of life's great challenges, from the heavy hitters like mortality, loss, and grief, right down to how not to get triggered by social media!

So, let us distil the lessons of the Stoics into a practical guide that this author has since adopted, with respect to dodging the cortisol bullet in daily life!

So, linking the learnings from the previous chapter, perceptions are king! And the perspectives of the Stoic greats like Marcus Aurelius, Seneca, and Epictetus were gems to combat accumulating or experiencing stress.

They use something that Delaney modified into being called the 'Control Test' to decide if something was worth stressing about. This test was simple to use and apply, and was simply qualifying matters as, in or out of our control. Then choosing to only adopt concern, worry, or stress about those items within our control.

THE CONTROL TEST

All that you can control is three things:

1. Your character
2. Your actions and reactions
3. How you treat others

The Stoics essentially eliminate 90% of modern sources of stress we get bombarded with daily by showing us we can release control of almost every single one of them as being out of our control.

Their guiding light to help steer us away from the murky waters of a stressful life is simple.

If it is out of our control, then it is not worth worrying about, precisely because it is out of our control!

This Control Test can be applied to any situation.

You are stressing if you will get the dream job you just applied for?

If the panel enjoyed your interview and found you suitable, it is out of your control.

If the company you are applying to work for is undergoing financial hardship and cuts the position last minute, this is out of your control.

Any multitude of factors could affect your chances of getting that dream job and almost none of them are within your control.

So, sleepless nights worrying and waiting by your phone for a call will do nothing but create needless stress in life, as the decision that you are giving control over your reality right now, is ironically not yours to control, to begin with!

If it isn't your character, actions, or how you treat someone, then release it.

Free your mind (and nervous system) from the burden of having to juggle the multitude of factors affecting your reality today that you have no control over!

This will be step one to releasing much of the anxiety of modern living.

If you come across a bad news story on your social media feed, what may have sent your cortisol sky-high previously could be diminished easily by asking:

Can I do anything about this right now through my actions, reactions, or how I treat others?

If the answer is no, then as tragic as that news story is, it's time to move on!

Apply the Stoic Control Test to any hurdle of contemporary living and watch the cortisol melt away!

OTHER STOIC LESSONS – RELATIVITY

When reading the journal of Marcus Aurelius in his 2000-year-old diary *Meditations*, I found strangely grounding words that would help anyone shift perspective on what is actually stressful.

The Stoics used the concept of '*memento mori*', which literally translated from Latin to 'remember that you die', to relativise their daily trials and tribulations.

When faced with insurmountable challenges, they would use intentional focus on their own mortality to realise that this challenge was nothing in the grand scheme of things.

When you consider that you have a finite time on this planet, you stop worrying about small details and start focusing on what matters. Living a life of meaning, being a person of great and resilient character, and acting in alignment with your values.

Anything outside of these powerful intentions and reflections was simply not worth losing sleep over.

Memento mori is a powerful tool to make you assess your current-day stresses against a much more pressing matter, your eventual exit from this mortal coil.

If you had the knowledge that you were going to die tomorrow, would what you fret about right now still seem significant and worth the stress you are giving to it?

If you realise your time is a ticking clock, does spending time stressing over being stuck in traffic or having a bad day at work really seem like your best use of mental resources?

Of course not.

We would realise almost everything we stress over is insignificant when we stack it against the looming reality of one's own mortality. It will make most hurdles seem insignificant and the stress will wash away like a weary tide upon the shores of reason.

It also would lend you a more logical perspective. One that dictates that there are actually some bigger picture things that are significant on the scale of mortality, that you should stress about.

That there actually are things you should be concerned with, but they are higher-order issues. Not just your current-day dramas.

Such matters, the Stoics considered worth worrying about were how to live a life of meaning, how to do good, and how to release the egotistic fuelled distractions of seeking status, fame, or wealth, and realise none of these materialistic concerns can be taken with us when we go.

So, only focus on what is a big enough impact, that if you stack it against the *Memento Mori* test, it still seems worth splitting hairs over!

DAILY RITUALS TO MAINTAIN
THIS GREAT HEADSPACE

We just did a bit of a deep dive on looking at the impacts of repressed emotional baggage and trauma as well as the power of relativity, by looking at some lessons from the Stoics to help us reframe what is actually stressful in the first place.

To be able to unpack our emotional baggage, or to think with a calm and rational mind required to think like the Stoics did, it requires a very clear, calm, and collected headspace.

You will not have a chance in hell of being able to think of the bigger picture, or use the Control Test, or analyse your own thoughts and how your childhood conditioning may be influencing your thoughts today, if your head is a scrambled, busy place!

So, to maintain a clear and level head, the author has come up with two simple, easy practices you can implement no matter where you are in the world, or how time-poor you are.

They are so simple, and easy to use, and make a MASSIVE difference to your headspace. They are two easy daily rituals:

1.   Journaling
2.   Walking Every Morning

JOURNALING

Now, a lot of folks make suggestions around their morning journaling that may feel like it has been turned into an academic or entrepreneurial enterprise, and not what it was intended to be.

People have been doing it for thousands of years, with amazing mental health benefits. Some of them have been a secret treasure chest of thoughts and dreams and hopes and goals, and for others, they have simply been a place to brain dump their daily lives in an attempt at maintaining sanity.

In rare instances, they have even become prolific works, with the personal journal of Marcus Aurelius *Memoirs* becoming a best-selling book still, even 2000 years after his death!

So, despite popular culture taking journaling and running with it, the way I encourage the reader to look at this suggestion of journaling is a much simpler exercise.

To maintain the clear headspace we spoke about earlier, I strongly recommend starting every morning by grabbing a pen and a piece of paper, before you do literally anything.

Don't check your phone, don't scroll social media, don't throw on the news.

Grab a pen and paper and find a quiet space that is nice and comfortable, and start to write down whatever is on your mind at the time.

I don't need you to write down your five-year plan, or your vision board, or to analyse your inner dialogues like some sort of Freudian understudy!

This is a super simple daily ritual whereby you just brain dump every single thing in your mind, on paper.

This will accomplish two things.

1. It will teach you to be an observer of your thoughts.
2. It will allow you to clear your mind and start the day with a clear and calm head.

It takes all of 10 minutes tops, and this exercise allows you to start paying attention to how much head noise you are carrying around with you on a daily basis.

A busy mind is a common handbrake and leads to a clouding of your ability to make calm and rational decisions.

Journaling will also allow you to start observing your thoughts and feelings and to identify patterns. As we spoke about in the section on psychology, observing our thoughts can point out recurring themes or areas we may wish to address, that are commonly affecting us in daily life.

If you are commonly fixated on an issue, or having some sort of habitual behaviour play out, you may not notice them in the busy day-to-day lives we lead.

But if you write them down every day and pay attention to what comes up regularly, you will have an excellent record of what behavioural loops, habits, or conditioning is playing out in your daily life.

So, in short, starting your day with a quick brain dump, where you just write down whatever is on your mind, will have a lot of benefits for you, the reader.

At the very least, you will walk away with a clear head and a note-pad full of ramblings, and best-case scenario, you will have a great resource of where to start in your next visit to your therapist!

WALKING EVERY MORNING

Now, walking as a form of exercise has amazing benefits in making us bulletproof to stress, that will be covered again in the physical habits section of this book.

However, for this section, we have recommended walking rather for the mental health benefits it can have, for clearing our mind and providing a space for peace and calm on a daily basis.

We all have so many commitments and stimuli in a normal day, that we could go days, week, or even months between finding opportunities for calmness.

Many people I have spoken to in my travels will report, the only occasions they feel peace in their lives is when they are on holidays from work, sprawled out on a beach chair somewhere, sipping cocktails.

This may only be once or twice a year for a lot of these people I speak to.

The problem with this is that if you don't make space for more times where you experience stillness and peace in your day, these may well be the only times you experience them.

This is very problematic for mental health.

Stillness is the essential ingredient for cultivating a calm mind.

A calm mind is the key tool we need to cope with daily stress.

The human brain was not designed to be drowned in stimulus 24/7 and if our day-to-day lives are a blur of texts, calls, emails, scrolling social media, binge watching Netflix, coffee, and a high-pressure job then it may well be that we only experience stillness and calm twice a year on that getaway with the hubby we spoke about!

If this sounds like you, it is no wonder we may have more head noise than we can bear.

And it makes perfect sense why you have a lot of mental chatter, when there is no space in your day for your mind to decompress. Right now, if your day sounds like how I described above, then creating a 20-minute space every morning as a daily ritual could be the most powerful tool you have to make you invulnerable to the stresses of daily living.

In a modern lifestyle full of 'input' in the form of stimulus, texts, calls, emails, scrolling socials, binging on TV, we need to create some time for 'output'.

We need to give ourselves a blissful window of tranquillity every morning to allow ourselves to decompress. I personally recommend doing this immediately after you have woken and journaled as well.

The feeling is amazing, starting every day with a clear mind from journaling then having a 20–30-minute walk with zero distractions, talking, calls, or phones.

I do this every day and it has been my most powerful tool in combatting the stresses of running a large business, with a dozen staff operating in multiple states, all whilst running podcasts, seminars, and workshops!

If I don't go on these walks and journal every morning, I notice myself becoming reactive. Becoming more impatient. Finding that my mind gets progressively busier.

Even last week, I skipped journaling and the walk for 3 days. I am human after all.

When I did my brain dump on day 4 and got back to journaling, I wrote three full A4 pages of handwritten scribble. My head felt like it was scrambled after 3 days of not journaling.

I couldn't maintain focus and my attention span was so short. I was snappy with colleagues.

After one morning back in the saddle, walking and journaling, I felt so much lighter and my head was so much clearer.

I highly recommend you give this a try for yourself.

For the next week, do this morning ritual every day and just brain dump everything you have in your head each morning upon rise.

Then go for a blissful walk and leave your phone behind.

No podcasts and no music. Just quiet, blissful walking. You can thank me later!

PHYSICAL INTERVENTIONS FOR NERVOUS SYSTEM REGULATION

Physical Exercise

Exercise is perceived by the body as a form of stress and stimulates the release of cortisol in kind.

In general, the more your fitness improves the better the body becomes at dealing with this physical stress.

This means that over time, less cortisol will be released during exercise and also in response to emotional or psychological stresses outside of the gym floor.

This is one proposed concept of how a stressful activity (like rigorous physical exercise) may make you better at dealing with stress long term, even if it spikes it in the short term!

In the realms of psychological benefits of exercise, another proposed concept of how exercise reduces stress long term is outlined here by an excerpt from a Harvard Health article:

'Regular aerobic exercise will bring remarkable changes to your body, your metabolism, your heart, and your spirits. It has a unique capacity to exhilarate and relax, to provide stimulation and calm, to counter depression and dissipate stress. It's a common experience among endurance athletes and has been verified in clinical trials that have successfully used exercise to treat anxiety disorders and clinical depression. If athletes and patients can derive psychological benefits from exercise, so can you.

How can exercise contend with problems as difficult as anxiety and depression? There are several explanations, some chemical, others behavioural.

The mental benefits of aerobic exercise have a neurochemical basis. Exercise reduces levels of the body's stress hormones, such as adrenaline and cortisol. It also stimulates the production of endorphins, chemicals in the brain that are the body's natural painkillers and mood elevators.' (24)

For the purpose of this book, we will look at how to approach exercise to improve your nervous system resilience.

There are a million benefits to exercise that we won't go in too deeply with this book, but what the author will set out to do is to give the reader a practical guide to customise what forms of exercise are most beneficial for cortisol management, when to exercise, and what to avoid when you are already stressed out!

FIRSTLY, TIMING IS EVERYTHING

Exercise is unique in that it is technically a short-term stressor on the body that long term leads to improved stress responses.

This is supported by studies, with this 2019 study finding that consistent exercise does indeed flatten the cortisol curve:

'We found a marked flattening of the diurnal cortisol slope...and a reduced cortisol at awakening...after 12 weeks of PE (Physical Exercise) treatment.' (25)

For those of you reading along at home, if you are interested in just how significantly cortisol was reduced from exercise, have a look at this graph from the study.

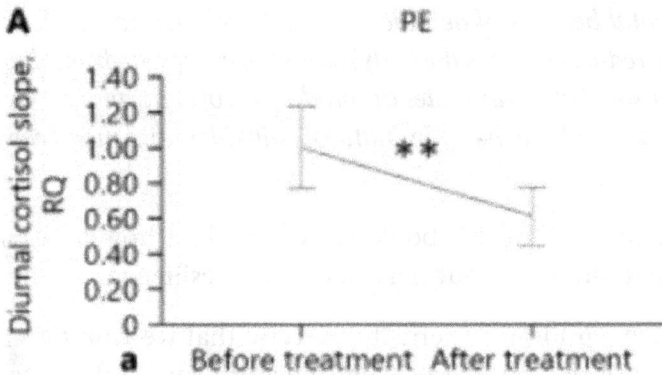

Figure 9 – Cortisol levels after 12 weeks of physical exercise (25).

Now, it may not appear much, but going from 1.0 before exercise was introduced to 0.6 after, it represents a 40% decrease in cortisol levels! That is massive!

This 2019 study further goes on to beautifully highlight that with consistent exercise, cortisol definitely is consistently lowered:

'On a neurobiological level, PE (physical exercise) modulates the hypothalamic-pituitary-adrenal axis, which is a part of the stress response system. Studies have shown that plasma cortisol levels are increased immediately after PE and that the plasma and urine cortisol levels decrease after repeated long-term PE' (25).

SO WHY ARE WE TALKING ABOUT TIMING RIGHT NOW?

Because, as this 2019 study highlights, exercise may lower stress in the long term, but in the short term, it actually increases cortisol!

Therefore, when planning our exercise routine, we need to be mindful that exercise often causes an acute cortisol increase, and it is therefore smart to plan our gym calendar with some priority around mornings vs evenings.

The author recommends mornings as the best time for intense exercise because, quite simply, it's working with your body and not against it when we structure it this way.

Cortisol naturally peaks in the morning and lowers in the evening.

So, if we know hard exercise will spike cortisol, we don't want to be placing it in the evening and interfering with the way nature designed our cortisol rhythm.

Intense exercise in the evenings would spike cortisol late in the day and therefore potentially interrupt sleep quality, leading to even more cortisol issues long term!

So, whether it is sprints, HIIT, heavyweight training, or your favourite CrossFit class, do your best to place your next workout in the mornings!

This is where the cortisol spike from the exercise will work synergistically with your body, as it is increasing cortisol at the time of the day our body naturally wants to!

Work with your body's natural rhythms and your cortisol levels will thank you!

EXERCISE SELECTION, INTENSITY, AND FREQUENCY TO MATCH YOUR STRESS LEVELS

The goal of this section is to give you a very practical assessment of how much exercise you can happily tolerate, and to also give you an insight into how to match exercise to your current stress levels.

Cortisol is a very catabolic hormone that, when elevated, will greatly reduce recovery, lead to muscle wastage, and make it hard to bounce back from hard workouts.

Simply put, if your nervous system is always jacked up with cortisol through the roof, placing additional physical demands in the form of exercise needs to be done very intentionally.

We need to look at the following when matching how much exercise you do, to your lifestyle:

1. Frequency (how often will you exercise?)
2. Modality (what types of exercise will you do?)
3. Intensity (how much and how hard will the exercise be?)

FREQUENCY

For those individuals in the high stress category, limiting intense exercise to 4 days per week is a great place to start.

For those with moderate stressors in their lives, 4–5 days in the gym is achievable whilst still maintaining recovery.

For those with low stress levels outside the weights room, you can more than likely head into the gym as often as you like!

MODALITY

High intensity rigorous exercises are the most impactful on acute cortisol levels.

High intensity exercises are those like weight lifting, HIIT work, metabolic training, sprints, and CrossFit.

These are the ones that are the heavy hitters, that are the meat and potatoes of most exercise routines, and do the most to change our fitness, body composition, and overall performance.

Think of these as the 'minimum effective dose' players that we use to build the foundations of your program.

They are the most bang for your buck, and give the greatest rewards physically, but if you are someone experiencing high stress in your life right now, be mindful of how much intense exercise you are currently doing.

The higher your stressors, the less intensity you can handle.

Next on the ladder is low and medium intensity exercise.

Medium intensity may be running, jogging, swimming, cycling, and other cardio activities.

Low Intensity refers more to walking, slow jogging, yoga, and Pilates.

As a rule of thumb, you can use the low intensity stuff as often as you please.

These exercise forms are often actually great for lowering mental stress and clearing the head, whilst having some great benefits for health.

The moderate intensity exercises we can add sparingly alongside the high intensity work, to increase aerobic fitness and metabolic health, but at the same time, they still impact recoverability and over all stress.

Moderate intensity exercise won't impact recovery nearly as much as high intensity exercise will, but it is still something to be added sparingly to assess your recoverability and stress levels in response to these activities.

INTENSITY

Intensity refers to the volume of work you intend to perform in your routine. In weight training, intensity is increased when we lift heavier weights or lift for more repetitions than previously.

In sprints, it may mean doing an additional 2 x 50 m dashes each week to build an aerobic base.

Whatever the exercise modality, intensity is how much we turn up the volume on how much of that exercise we perform in a week.

So, when planning an exercise routine to match your stress levels, being mindful of intensity is key.

High cortisol levels directly affect your ability to recover from intense exercise, and so, when considering intensity it must match your lifestyle and therefore your ability to recover.

WORKED EXAMPLE

What we mean by this is that the exercise program of a 19-year-old male who has no cares outside of a casual job at Bunnings and a weekend house party to plan is not what you would recommend to a high-level executive working 60-hour weeks whilst holding down a family.

These two individuals have wildly different demands on their time, and the mental stress load is wildly different.

The 19-year-old could likely engage in intense weight training 6 days a week, plus 5 km runs on weekends without running into too many issues.

His stress levels outside the gym are so minimal that even when buried in more volume in the weights room, he has the recover-ability to handle the workload because his cortisol levels would be very manageable outside of the training load.

Lower cortisol outside of the gym would make his ability to recover from training much higher and therefore he could hook into a high volume program and likely expect to reap the fruits of his labour!

The high-level executive working a 60-hour week, however, would already likely have sky-high cortisol most of his waking hours. He would also probably have less than optimal sleep with the kids at home, which as we know, will really drive stress levels skyward!

In sharp contrast to the teenager, even getting in 3–4 full body sessions at the gym a week would be about the most we can hope his nervous system could recover from, with all of the imposed demands outside of the gym floor.

His already high cortisol levels outside the weights room would mean he would have to be careful to train with a 'minimum effective dose' mentality, and be very wary about recoverability whilst stressors are high.

A PERSONAL CASE STUDY

I personally prescribe to the classification of a high stress individual, and can use my personal experience here to outline how someone may approach exercise.

When I started ramping up commitments with running my business, juggling a relationship, and starting to write this book, stress was at an all-time high. I was traditionally training 5 days a week for the last 10 years, so, it was all I knew!

But after taking stock of all of the stressors on my plate, I realised I no longer had the same recoverability of my 22-year-old, casually employed-self, being the director of a substantial business with a lot more plates to keep spinning!

So, I assessed my program.

I was doing 5 weight sessions with 5 exercises per session, doing 4 sets per exercise.

I was also finishing these workouts with 10 minutes on the treadmill doing minute on/minute off sprints.

I realised this was a massive volume to do in a week as an individual with very high lifestyle stressors.

So, I took my own advice and reduced from 5 weight sessions, that were followed by 10 minutes of HIIT daily to 4 days of weights per week, with the HIIT swapped for a 30-minute walk every morning.

The weights sessions went from 5 sessions/week, with 5 exercises x 4 sets per exercise each, to 4 sessions with 4 exercises per session, with only 3 sets per exercise.

I removed the HIIT all together and did my 30-minute walk at a gentle pace in the morning, as soon as I woke daily.

The difference was massive.

For the first time in forever, my weight started improving each week.

My dicky shoulder stopped having so many niggles.

I dropped some body fat off my stomach despite no changes in diet.

My libido returned (TMI maybe but this is a great metric for how much stress your body is under).

I had reduced my time in the gym 20% and was thriving!

All because I matched my exercise levels to my lifestyle.

SOME OTHER EXERCISE CONSIDERATIONS

Long-distance training, long bouts of weight training, or endurance training in general can lead to significant cortisol spikes above and beyond typical exercise.

This is a result of the length of the exercise, more so than the type of exercise itself.

Exercising over 60 minutes can lead to marked increases in cortisol, which will further hamper recovery, promote muscle wastage, and leave us in a catabolic state.

Therefore, as one final consideration, when matching your exercise to the stressors in your lifestyle, keep lengthy gym or running sessions out of your program if you have high stress floating around.

It is best to keep bouts over 60 minutes for when your nervous system is resilient and well-rested and lifestyle stressors are under control!

BREATHWORK

Breathwork, also known as controlled or intentional breathing exercises, is a technique that involves consciously manipulating your breath to influence your physical and mental state.

When it comes to reducing cortisol and stress levels, breathwork can be quite effective due to several physiological and psychological mechanisms. Here's how it works:

1. **Activation of the Parasympathetic Nervous System**: Breathwork, particularly deep and slow breathing, stimulates the parasympathetic nervous system. This is the 'rest-and-digest' mode of your autonomic nervous system, responsible for promoting relaxation and reducing stress. When activated, it counteracts the 'fight-or-flight' response triggered by the sympathetic nervous system, which is associated with increased cortisol production.

2. **Reducing Hyperventilation**: In stressful situations, people often experience shallow and rapid breathing (hyperventilation), leading to an imbalance of oxygen and carbon dioxide levels in the body. Breathwork encourages deeper and slower breathing, helping to restore the balance of these gases. This can prevent overstimulation of the sympathetic nervous system and lower cortisol levels.

3. **Mindfulness and Meditation**: Many breathwork techniques involve mindfulness and meditation practices. Focusing on your breath and being present in the moment can help redirect your thoughts away from stressors and anxious thinking. This mental shift contributes to a reduction in cortisol and stress.

4. **Altering Heart Rate Variability (HRV)**: Certain breathwork practices such as coherent breathing, can positively impact heart rate variability (HRV). HRV refers to the variation in time between successive heartbeats, and higher HRV is associated with better stress resilience. Breathwork can enhance HRV, leading to reduced cortisol levels and a more relaxed state.

5. **Release of Endorphins**: Some breathwork techniques, like breath of fire in yoga, are thought to activate the release of endorphins, natural feel-good chemicals in the brain. Endorphins help to counteract stress and promote feelings of well-being.

6. **Improved Oxygenation and Blood Flow**: By consciously controlling your breath, you can enhance oxygen delivery to tissues and improve blood circulation. This can reduce physical tension and promote a sense of relaxation, which in turn lowers stress and cortisol levels.

BREATHWORK TECHNIQUES TO REDUCE STRESS

There are several common breathwork practices that can help lower cortisol and stress levels. These techniques are simple and can be easily incorporated into your daily routine. Here are some effective ones:

1. **Deep Belly Breathing (Diaphragmatic Breathing)**:

- Find a comfortable sitting or lying position.
- Place one hand on your chest and the other on your abdomen.
- Inhale deeply through your nose, expanding your diaphragm, and feeling your abdomen rise.
- Exhale slowly through your mouth, allowing your abdomen to fall.
- Focus on the sensation of your breath and repeat for several minutes.

2. **4-7-8 Breathing**:

- Sit or lie down in a relaxed position.
- Inhale through your nose for a count of 4.
- Hold your breath for a count of 7.
- Exhale slowly and completely through your mouth for a count of 8.
- Repeat this cycle for a few minutes.

3. **Box Breathing (Square Breathing)**:

- Sit comfortably and inhale deeply through your nose for a count of 4.
- Hold your breath for a count of 4.
- Exhale slowly through your mouth for a count of 4.

- Hold your breath again for a count of 4.
- Repeat the process for several rounds.

4. Coherent Breathing:

- Sit or lie down comfortably.
- Inhale slowly and deeply through your nose for a count of 6.
- Exhale slowly and completely through your nose for a count of 6.
- Aim to maintain a steady and equal duration for both the inhale and exhale.
- Continue for at least 5–10 minutes.

Find the techniques that resonate best with you and incorporate them into your daily routine. Consistency is key, and practicing these techniques regularly can help you manage stress, reduce cortisol levels, and promote a sense of calm and relaxation. If you're new to breathwork, consider seeking guidance from a certified breathwork instructor to ensure you're using proper techniques, and to tailor the practice to your specific needs.

ICE BATHS AND COLD WATER IMMERSION.

This is a new field of emerging study, with CWI and ice baths being the hot topic in the fitness community in recent times.

Ice baths and cold water immersion (CWI) are known to have a multitude of benefits for lowering inflammation, improving metabolic health, increasing insulin sensitivity, fat loss, and reduction in stress and mood disorders (22). This is backed by the 2022 meta-analysis:

'Ice bathing has been suggested to have many health benefits. For example, in the popular literature it has been claimed that it can boost the immune system, treat depression, enhance peripheral circulation, increase libido, burn calories and reduce stress' (22).

Interestingly, the data shows profound changes in chemistry when looking at adrenaline, cortisol, metabolic rate, and dopamine levels after exposure (23):

'To differentiate between the effect of cold (immersion) on hormone and cardiovascular functions of man, a group of young men was examined during 1-h head-out immersions in water of different temperatures (32 degrees C, 20 degrees C and 14 degrees C). Immersion in water at 32 degrees C did not change rectal temperature and metabolic rate, but lowered heart rate (by 15%) and systolic and diastolic blood pressures (by 11 %, or 12%, respectively), compared to controls at ambient air temperature... cortisol and aldosterone concentrations were also lowered (by 46%, 34%, and 17%, respectively...

Cold water immersion (14 degrees C) lowered rectal temperature and increased metabolic rate (by 350%), heart rate and systolic and diastolic blood pressure (by 5%, 7%, and 8%, respectively). Plasma noradrenaline and dopamine concentrations were increased by 530% and by 250% respectively...'

These findings are wild!

The 14-degree water is nowhere near ice bath territory. In fact, the ocean is often at around these temps in winter!

This study showed, that an hour in cold water dropped cortisol by 46%, increased metabolic rate by 350%, and lowered blood pressure by 15%. This is insanely great for health!

After finding such powerful findings from CWI or ice baths, the author started investigating what pathways ice baths and CWI activate, which may explain how they can benefit your nervous system so tremendously!

Interestingly, the data suggested that ice baths and CWI actually seem to increase cortisol secretion acutely, and demonstrated elevated cortisol and epinephrine levels after exposures to ice baths specifically.

So, for those of you reading along at home, your inner dialogue may look a little something like this at this stage of the chapter:

'Well, if ice baths increase stress hormones, how does that help me become more resilient to stress? I don't want more stress, I am trying to limit it!'

There are two possible mechanisms that may make ice baths and CWI beneficial for stress.

One is stimulating the vagus nerve to modulate the nervous system.

The second is via activation of the sirtuins.

Experiencing these extreme events, like very low temperature exposure, activates the vagus nerve through the dermis (skin) and causes immediate responses to protect from the stress, that are beneficial for overall health.

The vagus nerve is a long nerve that runs from your brain to your stomach.

It's responsible for a variety of functions, such as controlling your heart rate, blood pressure, and stress response.

When you're stressed, the vagus nerve signals your body to release stress hormones.

When you take an ice bath, the cold water has a calming effect that activates the vagus nerve to decrease stress levels and to help reduce tension and anxiety.

Cold exposure influences the vagus nerve to initially activate the sympathetic nervous system, in an effort to maintain body temperatures.

Whilst this is a short-term spike in stress, it then leads to a compensatory parasympathetic activation in the following hours that balances out the spike.

The best way to foster resilience is by building a nervous system that can be activated and then brought down to a regular state, as fast as possible.

CWI and ice baths are deliberate imposed stresses that our nervous system then overcompensates and goes into hyperdrive activating parasympathetic pathways immediately, in an effort to return to normal after these extreme cold exposures.

In doing so, this slingshot back towards parasympathetic makes us more resilient to future stressors, as our nervous system practises going from acute stress back to rest-and-digest.

The second potential concept that stress on the body can be beneficial in activating protective and beneficial responses, really leans into an area coined 'hormesis' by Dr. David Sinclair.

Dr. David Sinclair is one of the leading researchers on how stressors can enhance longevity and lifespan currently, via sirtuin activation.

This body of research is all around how imposing deliberate stressors on the body can stimulate the sirtuins and stress-related pathways to kick-start beneficial biological processes.

Whether it is sirtuin activation, vagus nerve modulation, or some other yet-to-be-explored pathways that make ice baths and CWI great, one thing is clear from the data.

Ice baths and CWI lower cortisol, blood pressure, and anxiety when implemented regularly!

NUTRITION

'While a healthy diet is often recommended as a strategy for managing stress and stress-related diseases, there are no evidence-based, specific dietary guidelines that target such concerns. There is a growing awareness about the advantages of nutritional medicine in psychiatry, prompting an increased focus on the interrelationships between stress, mood, and nutrition' (18).

This is an excerpt from a 2019 study looking specifically to find the effects that certain nutritional interventions have on cortisol and stress levels, and it perfectly summarises the intent of this chapter of the book.

It is common knowledge that a healthy diet is a powerful lever to pull in the war on stress management.

But to give you, the reader, more specifics than just saying 'eat healthy', we have unpacked the literature and found some very specific actionable nutritional strategies that can directly lower stress levels in your life!

MAIN NUTRITIONAL INTERVENTIONS WE WILL EXPLORE INCLUDE:

→ The protective effects of carbs/insulin on cortisol levels

→ The effects of consuming carbs pre- / post-workout on cortisol levels

→ The protective effects EPA/DHEA have against stress and their effect on the brain

→ Not having caffeine on an empty stomach and eliminating alcohol

INSULIN AND CORTISOL – THE TALE OF TWO ANTAGONISTS

Negative feedback loops exist all over biology.

These feedback loops are our body's innate check and balancing system, whereby there are naturally opposing hormones, enzymes, processes, and pathways that work in perfectly opposed unison to keep the body in homeostasis.

When one pathway is driven hard, another backs off to compensate.

Stress is not immune to these biological feedback loops!

So, when trying to understand how nutrition fits into the bigger picture of making you bulletproof to stress, we need to understand one key loop.

This loop is the antagonistic relationship between cortisol and insulin.

Understanding of this feedback loop with cortisol and insulin will allow us to deploy specific nutritional strategies, that can take advantage of one such negative feedback loop in our favour to help regulate our nervous system, and get stress under wraps!

Insulin is a storage hormone and a very anabolic one to boot!

Whenever we eat something containing carbohydrates, our body breaks that down into simple units of glucose (sugar), and this then enters the bloodstream to be transported where it is needed.

Blood sugar is regulated by the pancreas.

In response to increases in blood sugar, the pancreas secretes the powerful hormone insulin, which is responsible for keeping this blood sugar in a very tight range.

The insulin then regulates blood sugar by shuttling the blood sugar off to the muscles to store as glycogen. This will become our energy reserves that we will call upon when our muscles need quick fuel to burn!

Now the other useful function of insulin is that it is a driver of pathways that are the polar opposite to those that cortisol activate.

Cortisol is a catabolic hormone. A catabolic state is the opposite to an anabolic one, which is where our body is building, growing, and repairing.

A high cortisol and catabolic state is one that breaks things down.

Imagine when your cortisol is high, it is like your body is having a fire sale, desperately trying to clear stock to get some quick cash together! That cash represents energy, and cortisol will try to break down anything it can to get fuel into the system to fuel 'flight-or-fight'.

So, where does nutrition come into this conversation?

Well, simply put, if we know that being stressed out and in flight/ fight is catabolic, and insulin is a hormone that is anabolic, here lies a great opportunity to use food to moderate stress!

When insulin is high, cortisol is lowered.

Carbohydrate containing foods increase blood sugar.

Increased blood sugar increases insulin secretion, thus blunting cortisol levels.

So, if we are trying to manage stress in the body, the best thing we can do is keep some healthy carbohydrate rich meals in our diet to keep insulin around, thus keeping cortisol levels under wraps throughout the day.

This is summarised perfectly in the 2019 study excerpt (18):

'In support of this finding, we also found significant (P < 0.05) and inverse linear associations between dietary carbohydrate and… salivary cortisol(levels), with the strongest negative association occurring at 30 min post-TSST (Trier Social Stress Test, TSST).'

This study looked at the effects a higher carb diet has on stress levels.

Now there are specific times this is more beneficial than others.

We also need to be mindful that we can't just have a candy bar every time we are stressed! Moderation is key with insulin, especially in a time when type 2 diabetes and metabolic diseases are running rampant in western society!

But it is a powerful tool to utilise!

It also explains why we experience more stress when dieting, to a certain extent.

As we covered earlier in the book, being in calorie deficit in itself increased cortisol secretion significantly. But what do most people cut first when dieting?

Carbs!

The words 'low carb' and 'dieting' are two peas in a pod for most of the everyday dieters! The author would hazard a guess that the vast majority of people who start a diet begin by cutting carbs.

This hasn't been helped by the recent crazes around ketogenic dieting, which demonised carbohydrates in recent years.

In fact, high-fat/low-carb dieting has massive effects on cortisol, as seen in the 2019 study (18) which found:

'high-fat feeding increases circulating corticosterone in rodent models and high-fat meals were shown to exacerbate detrimental autonomic nervous systems and cardiovascular responses to stress'.

Now, these are murky waters to debate because the food pyramid for western society since 2011 has recommended that our diet should be at least 50% carbohydrates. This has become a disaster for the vast majority of the largely sedentary, non-exercising general population.

Obesity, insulin resistance, and metabolic diseases are rampant now thanks to this extremist skew of macronutrients towards carbohydrates.

So, it is not the mission of this chapter to say every meal should be served atop a bed of white rice.

But it is worthy of note for anyone embarking on a dieting phase, or who are interested in pursuing a lower carb diet, or exploring the benefits of ketogenic dieting, to beware that carbs have a very protective effect on cortisol.

Removing the majority of carbs from our diet may be a bad idea if we have a lot of stress in our lives as having these carbohydrate containing meals would allow us to leverage insulin's powerful negative feedback loop with cortisol!

So, how do we best utilise carbohydrates in our nutrition to keep our cortisol levels under wraps?

I would advise using them strategically.

There are a few key times we can consume carbohydrates and get the most bang for our buck with insulin, and those times are:

1.   Pre- or Post-Exercise Carbohydrate Consumption

Consuming carbs pre- and/or post-workout is a very simple and powerful intervention that I have deployed with a lot of clients as well as myself and noticed massive benefits.

For the morning trainers, it has a specific benefit of giving your body a ready fuel source after 8 hours of sleeping, with no fuel to burn.

Sleep is for all intents and purposes, a fasting window.

So, anyone who does the old 'rise and grind' and trains in the morning as soon as they wake up, would really benefit from some high glycaemic carbohydrates prior to working out. Especially if the workout is intense such as weightlifting or sprints.

As a rule of thumb for athletic individuals, 30–60 grams of carbs per 60 minutes of exercise is recommended (16) depending on body weight and intensity of the training.

It is also recommended to have between 0.7 g/kg–1 g/kg of body weight of carbohydrates within an hour of finishing this intense exercise, to ensure replenishment of spent muscle and liver's glycogen stores (16) and maintenance of stable blood sugar levels.

For less athletic individuals, the post-workout meal isn't as essential, but we definitely would like to see a good pre-workout meal consumed 1 hour before training, with 30–60 g of carbohydrates for each hour of training you have planned.

This will maximise performance and significantly stabilise blood sugar levels, which is also critical for managing cortisol levels.

This nutritional strategy of consuming a higher carbohydrate intake around exercise to lower cortisol is heavily backed by science as well (17).

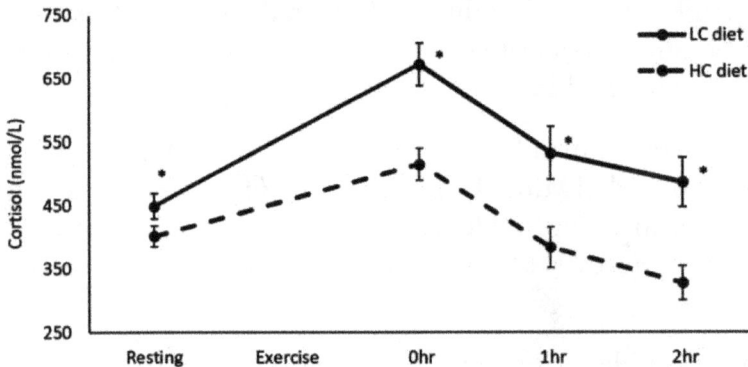

Figure 10 – Resting, 0 h, 1 h, and 2 h post-exercise cortisol after long-duration exercise, on short-term low carb (LC) vs higher carb (HC) diets. Carbohydrate consumption significantly reduced cortisol levels for hours after training (17).

This figure shows a nearly 50% increase in post-workout cortisol levels on a lower carbohydrate diet vs a higher carbohydrate diet. This demonstrates clearly, the powerful effects carbohydrates have on lowering stress on the body, especially for those exercising regularly!

2.   Before Bed

Dr. Alan Christianson is a naturopathic medical doctor and author of the book *The Adrenal Reset Diet*.

This excerpt from his book, summarises perfectly why carbohydrate consumption in the evening is ideal for stress management and particularly optimising sleep quality in the process. He also gives a good summary of how carbs can be used strategically to modulate cortisol throughout the day.

'So, the idea is by having a lower carb breakfast, you can sustain higher morning cortisol, which is desirable to a point. You cannot

elevate an appropriate cortisol level, but you can allow it to move to a good range if it's suppressed.

At midday, cortisol is basically neutral, so you intake a moderate amount of carbs. What we are doing at this point is supporting the gradual reduction of cortisol.

In the evening, you are enjoying a meal higher in good, healthy carbs. The idea with this is we are supporting the appropriate shutdown of cortisol, which allows you good, restorative sleep. (It turns out that quality sleep may be a bigger factor for long-term weight loss than even diet or exercise.) If you simply avoid carbs, sleep quality suffers.

When you don't eat enough carbs in the evening to go deeper into sleep, your body gets hypoglycaemic. Your body needs glucose for your brain and muscles to function. You'll make glucose by breaking down your muscles, and you need cortisol to do this. So, when you're too low in your carbs, you raise cortisol, pull your muscles apart, and make glucose out of that. When this happens, your cortisol level elevates higher than it should. This is a real problem in the evening.'

This is a great explanation of how we can leverage the relationship of cortisol and insulin to better modulate stress levels in the body and in doing so, making our nervous system healthier long term.

Particularly in the evening, it is beneficial to have carbohydrates around to lower cortisol, allowing a greater sleep quality.

It is, however, important these are a low glycaemic carb, like pumpkin, sweet potato, whole grains, or wholemeal pasta. High GI carbs may have the opposite effects on sleep quality because there will definitely be an insulin spike, but it will be sharp. You run the risk of there being a corresponding low in blood sugar too with a high GI carb, and as we have covered, the low blood sugar will often use cortisol to liberate the blood sugar our body wants stable. So, opt for low GI carb sources before bed, and you will get all the pros and none of the cons of insulin around bedtime!

THE PROTECTIVE EFFECTS OF FATTY ACIDS (EPA/DHA) AGAINST STRESS

We just deep dived into everything to do with insulin and cortisol, and how carbs can be leveraged strategically to lower cortisol.

We will now look at the role essential fatty acids (EFAs) have on stress levels!

There is some great data out there on how the EFA-rich Mediterranean diet is amazing for cardiovascular health, inflammation, and heart disease. There are also mountains of research on fish oil and its amazing benefits.

This chapter is concerned with how we can deploy dietary fats, specifically supplementation with fish oil, to moderate stress.

This diagram demonstrates a powerful effect on long-term supplementation of the fats, olive oil as well as fish oil on perceived stress. As the study, this diagram came from, can attest, both olive and fish oil really did help lower perceived stress levels (19).

MEASURE: PSS Perceived Stress Scale

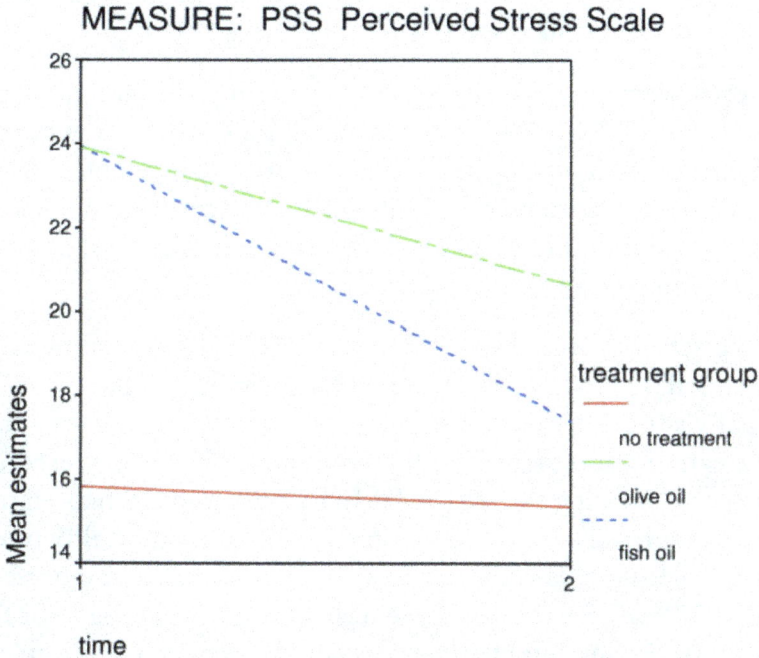

Figure 11 – This diagram demonstrates a powerful effect on long term supplementation of the fats, olive oil as well as fish oil on perceived stress levels

This study actually refers to the effects of fish oil as being somewhat 'adaptogenic' to stress.

I wanted to explore what pathways may be driven by the omega-3 supplementation in reducing stress levels, so I started trawling the literature.

There were mountains of data on omega-3s lowering inflammation, with inflammation being a well-known stressor in the body. The inflammation dampening effects of fish oil supplementation may well be a primary pathway in how they help reduce stress on the body.

Alternatively, positive changes in body composition that occur as a result of fish oil supplementation, may also be a factor in why stress is lowered when omegas are supplemented with. This is explored further in the ISSN study excerpt below, where it was found that cortisol levels lowered when fish oil supplementation was introduced (20).

'In conclusion, 6 weeks of supplemental fish oil significantly increased lean mass, and significantly reduced fat mass in healthy adults... The reduction in salivary cortisol following fish oil treatment was significantly correlated with the increased fat free mass and the decreased fat mass observed... Since higher salivary cortisol levels are associated with higher mortality rates, the reduction in salivary cortisol levels observed in the present study following fish oil supplementation likely has significant implications beyond positive changes in body composition.'

This highlights that EFA supplementation with omega-3s improved body composition, and in so doing, likely explained the consequent lowering of circulating cortisol levels.

There were also significant benefits to omega-3 supplementation in those with chronically high stress (21).

This excerpt from the 2012 study concluded:

'Nutrients such as omega-3 oils and phosphatidylserine have been considered to exert stress-buffering effects. In this randomised, double-blind, placebo-controlled trial, we investigated effects of omega-3 phosphatidylserine (PS) on perceived chronic stress, assessed by the Trier Inventory for Chronic Stress, and on *psychobiological stress responses to an acute laboratory stress protocol, the Trier Social Stress Test (TSST)...*

'We hypothesized that omega-3 PS supplementation lowers chronic and acute stress...By accounting for chronic stress level of study participants, stress-reducing effects of omega-3 PS were found exclusively for high chronically stressed subjects. As expected, these individuals also showed a blunted cortisol response to the Trier Social Stress Test. Treatment with omega-3 PS seemed to restore the cortisol response in this particular subgroup of low responders. These results are in line with previous findings. We conclude that subgroups characterized by high chronic stress and/ or a dysfunctional response of the hypothalamus-pituitary-adrenal axis may profit from omega-3 PS supplementation.'

What we are shown by these findings is that 12 weeks of supplementing with fish oil helped restore normal cortisol responses in chronically stressed study participants. This could represent another excellent pathway, that omega 3s seem to buffer the body from the negative effects of stress!

After a thorough deep dive into the literature on the topic, it is the recommendation of the author that anyone reading along at home would benefit by supplementing with 4000 mg of fish oil per day (containing approx. 1600 mg of EPA/DHA).

This supplement would be a great idea for those looking to further lower perceived stress, reduce inflammation, and improve body composition!

It would also be wise to include a decent amount of healthy essential fatty acids into your diet daily from sources, such as olive oil, nuts, seeds, and oily fish.

This will help dampen inflammation and perceived stress and improve body composition long term.

FASTED CAFFEINE CONSUMPTION AND ELIMINATING ALCOHOL

The consumption of caffeine upon the rise can have a massive effect on the CAR.

CAR refers to cortisol awakening response, which is the tracking of cortisol secretion in the first part of the day and upon the rise, specifically to monitor the health of your nervous system.

As we established in Part 1 of the book, cortisol is naturally at its peak within 1 hour of waking daily. This is also coincidentally when most people prefer to have their morning coffee.

Now, this will definitely drive cortisol to be on the higher side of optimal, being that caffeine is a CNS stimulant and can lead to elevated cortisol. This is problematic as it may exacerbate existing stress and anxiety throughout the day, and more troublingly, lead to more cortisol secretion later in the day due to the relationship between caffeine, blood sugar, and Cortisol.

When caffeine is consumed upon rising before eating breakfast, we are in a low blood sugar and peak cortisol state. This means the extra caffeine will ramp up cortisol, whilst the low blood sugar in the presence of stimulants will also lead the body to use cortisol to liberate stored fuel to get available blood sugar to burn. It's a double attack on stress!

To prevent this, having a meal with some complex carbohydrates to stabilise blood sugar before having your morning coffee, will ensure that your low blood sugar combined with stimulants won't make your body secrete cortisol to get sugar into the blood.

This is a big problem for those who practise intermittent fasting as well.

Those who caffeinate during these fasting windows, again with low blood sugar and no present fuel source (i.e., food) available, set themselves up for a cortisol fiesta!

Every time our body senses low blood sugar accompanied by a sensed demand for energy (like when you consume caffeine), then it will use cortisol to liberate stored fuel and dump it into the bloodstream. The relationship between insulin, blood sugar, and cortisol is well documented earlier in this chapter.

So, to best buffer yourself against one of the most common cortisol sources, try and consume caffeine 90 minutes after rising, and preferably never on an empty stomach, or when fasting.

Also, moderate your total caffeine intake in your diet to no more than 2–3 mg of caffeine per kg of body weight. For example, a 100 kg male should keep caffeine to 200–300 mg daily.

ELIMINATE ALCOHOL

We cover alcohol extensively in Chapter 1 of the book, as a common source of stress for a lot of people.

Ironically, despite being the most common source of stress relief for much of society, it is also an acute stressor on the body, that leads to deterioration in sleep quality, and increased perceived stress, throughout the days following alcohol consumption.

Because we covered alcohol extensively earlier in the book, we won't go into great depth here.

Instead, we will simply make a science-backed recommendation to eliminate alcohol from your diet as much as humanly possible. We are all human, and yes, alcohol is a big part of social circles in many cultural groups. So, there are more factors to consider, but if you are serious in your quest to give your nervous system a breather from stress, then limiting alcohol to as close to zero as possible, will do you wonders!

INTRODUCE ADRENAL SUPPLEMENTATION

Adrenal supplements describe products that support or improve the function of the adrenal glands, which, as we know, are the glands responsible for producing hormones, such as cortisol and adrenaline.

These supplements often contain a combination of vitamins, minerals, and herbal extracts that are believed to nourish and support the adrenal glands.

The idea behind using adrenal supplements to lower stress is based on the following mechanisms:

1. **Cortisol Regulation:** Cortisol is a hormone produced by the adrenal glands in response to stress. It plays a significant role in the body's fight-or-flight response. Adrenal supplements may contain ingredients that are thought to help regulate cortisol levels. By supporting healthy cortisol production, these supplements aim to prevent excessive cortisol spikes that can occur during times of chronic stress.

2. **Nutrient Support:** Adrenal supplements often contain vitamins and minerals that are important for adrenal gland function. These may include vitamin C, B vitamins (especially B5 and B6), magnesium, and zinc, among others. Providing these nutrients in adequate amounts may help optimise adrenal function, potentially reducing stress, and supporting overall well-being.

3. **Adaptogenic Herbs:** Some adrenal supplements include adaptogenic herbs, which are believed to help the body adapt to stress and maintain balance. Examples of adaptogens that are commonly included in these supplements include ashwagandha, *Rhodiola rosea*, eleuthero (Siberian ginseng), and holy basil. These herbs are thought to modulate the body's stress response, leading to a reduction in stress and cortisol levels.

4. **Energy and Fatigue:** Chronic stress can lead to fatigue and exhaustion, which may impact overall well-being. Adrenal supplements often contain ingredients that are believed to support energy levels and combat fatigue. These ingredients may include coenzyme Q10, D-ribose, or certain amino acids.

Many of these supplements are listed with appropriate dosages in Part 1 of the book and are an excellent tool to implement into your daily routine when looking to become bulletproof to stress.

The best place to start is to look for a quality company who makes an adrenal supplement containing the herbs at the dosages you will find in the early pages of this book.

Ashwagandha, L-Theanine, holy basil, and lemon balm are amongst my favourites to include and feature in the adrenal product I formulated under my supplement company.

Taking this category of supplements before bed is my recommendation, as when taken at this time, these supplements will greatly improve sleep quality, lower perceived stress, reduce time taken to get to sleep, and increase mood, energy levels, and libido throughout the day.

They can also be used throughout the day at lower doses (for example, I love to use 600 mg of ashwagandha before bed for better sleep, or 200–300 mg during the day when I have a full-on day at work to lower perceived stress).

When used during the day, adaptogenic herbs help us adapt to our environment and become more resilient to stressors. They are nature's tools to help us fight the deleterious effects of stress on the body.

For a beginner stack before bed, try:

- 600 mg Ashwagandha (std. to 5% Withanolides)
- 100 mg L-Theanine
- 500 mg Lemon Balm
- 500 mg Holy Basil
- 100 mg Passion Flower Extract

This will greatly reduce stress before bed and increase sleep quality markedly.

THE TAKE HOME

IF YOU HAVE read along this far, thank you for taking the time to learn every single facet of how we can better deal with stress in our daily lives.

In Part 1, we looked at common sources of stress, how our body functions when under stress, and how it looks when it goes wrong!

Part 2 is then a practical guide showing both mental, psychological, and physical interventions you can start as of tomorrow, to make yourself bulletproof to stress.

Through consistent implementation of some or all of these practises, hopefully, you, the reader, will walk away with something of immense value on your quest to becoming bulletproof to stress!

It has become a personal mission of the author for nearly a decade now, to help educate people on the impact of stress on their hormones, sleep, daily lives, and quality of life.

By reading along at home, you have helped me achieve this mission of creating a positive impact on a large scale by spreading awareness about the silent killer of our nervous system and quality of life!

Thank you for reading, and I sincerely hope this book has represented something of value to you all!

REFERENCE LIST

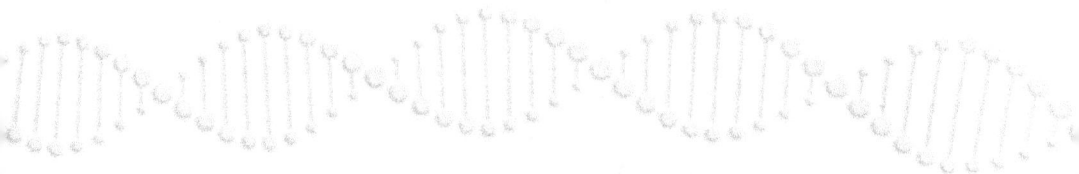

SCIENTIFIC LITERATURE
REFERENCE MATERIAL

Tindle J, Tadi P. Neuroanatomy, Parasympathetic Nervous System. StatPearls [Internet]. 2020 Jan 11Available from:.https://www.statpearls.com/articlelibrary/viewarticle/26653/ (accessed 30.1.2021)

Robert L. Spencer, Ph.D., and Kent E. Hutchison, Ph.D., Journal of Alcohol Research and Health, Vol. 23, No. 4, 1999

(1A) Chu B, Marwaha K, Sanvictores T, et al. Physiology, Stress Reaction. [Updated 2022 Sep 12].

Hirotsu C, Tufik S, Andersen ML. Interactions between sleep, stress, and metabolism: From physiological to pathological conditions. Sleep Sci. 2015 Nov

Pincomb GA, Lovallo WR, McKey BS, Sung BH, Passey RB, Everson SA, Wilson MF. Acute blood pressure elevations with caffeine in men with borderline systemic hypertension. *Am J Cardiol.* 1996;77:270–4.

Lovallo WR, Whitsett TL, al'Absi M, Sung BH, Vincent AS, Wilson MF. Caffeine stimulation of cortisolsecretion across the waking hours in relation to caffeine intake levels. Psychosom Med. 2005 Sep-Oct;67(5):734-9.

Lovallo WR, Al'Absi M, Blick K, Whitsett TL, Wilson MF. Stress-like adrenocorticotropin responses to caffeine in young healthy men. Pharmacol Biochem Behav. 1996 Nov;55

Working Time Arrangements, Australia, November 2009 (cat. no. 6342.0), Australian Bureau of Statistics.

Faraut B, Bayon V, Léger D. Neuroendocrine, immune and oxidative stress in shift workers. Sleep Med Rev. 2013

Bostock S, Steptoe A. Influences of early shift work on the diurnal cortisolrhythm, mood and sleep: within-subject variation in male airline pilots. Psychoneuroendocrinology. 2013;38:533–541

Manenschijn L, van Kruysbergen RG, de Jong FH, Koper JW, van Rossum EF. Shift work at young age is associated with elevated long-term cortisollevels and body mass index. J Clin Endocrinol Metab. 2011;96

Weibel L, Spiegel K, Follenius M, Ehrhart J, Brandenberger G. Internal dissociation of the circadian markers of the cortisolrhythm in night workers. Am J Phys. 1996

Li J, Bidlingmaier M, Petru R, Pedrosa Gil F, Loerbroks A, Angerer P. Impact of shift work on the diurnal cortisolrhythm: a one-year longitudinal study in junior physicians. J Occup Med Toxicol. 2018 Aug 14;13:23.

Lopresti AL. The Effects of Psychological and Environmental Stress on Micronutrient Concentrations in the Body: A Review of the Evidence. Adv Nutr. 2020 Jan 1;11

Yasmin F, Haleem DJ, Haleem MA. Effects of repeated restraint stress on serum electrolytes in ethanol-treated and water-treated rats. Pak J Pharm Sci. 2007 Jan

(14A) Ogden CL, Carroll MD, Curtin LR, McDowell MA, Tabak CJ, Flegal KM. Prevalence of overweight and obesity in the United States, 1999 –2004. JAMA 2006; 295:1549 –55.

(14B) Centres for Disease Control and Prevention. National Health and Nutrition Examination Survey Data. Hyattsville, MD: National Center for Health Statistics; 2009.

A. J. Tomiyama et al. 'Low Calorie Dieting Increases Cortisol'. Psychosomatic Medicine 72:000 – 000 (2010).

Hassapidou M. 'Carbohydrate requirements of elite athletes'. British Journal of Sports Medicine 2011;45:e2.

Whittaker J, Harris M. Low-carbohydrate diets and men's cortisoland testosterone: Systematic review and meta-analysis. Nutr Health. 2022 Dec;28(4):543-554. doi: 10.1177/02601060221083079. Epub 2022 Mar 7. Erratum in: Nutr Health. 2022 Dec;28(4):783. PMID: 35254136; PMCID: PMC9716400.

Soltani H, Keim NL, Laugero KD. Increasing Dietary Carbohydrate as Part of a Healthy Whole Food Diet Intervention Dampens Eight Week Changes in Salivary Cortisoland Cortisol Cortisoleness. Nutrients. 2019 Oct 24;11(11):2563. doi: 10.3390/nu11112563. PMID: 31652899; PMCID: PMC6893582.

Bradbury J, Myers SP, Oliver C. An adaptogenic role for omega-3 fatty acids in stress; a randomised placebo-controlled double-blind intervention study (pilot) [ISRCTN22569553]. Nutr J. 2004 Nov 28;3:20. doi: 10.1186/1475-2891-3-20. PMID: 15566625; PMCID: PMC538287.

Noreen, Eric E. et al Effects of supplemental fish oil on resting metabolic rate, body composition, and salivary cortisolin healthy adults. Journal of the International Society of Sports Nutrition.

Juliane Hellhammer, Torsten Hero, Nadin Franz, Carina Contreras, Melanie Schubert, Omega-3 fatty acids administered in phosphatidylserine improved certain aspects of high chronic stress in men, Nutrition Research, Volume 32, Issue 4, 2012,

Esperland D, de Weerd L, Mercer JB. Health effects of voluntary exposure to cold water – a continuing subject of debate. Int J Circumpolar Health. 2022 Dec;81(1):2111789. doi: 10.1080/22423982.2022.2111789. PMID: 36137565; PMCID: PMC9518606.

Srámek P, Simecková M, Janský L, Savlíková J, Vybíral S. Human physiological responses to immersion into water of different temperatures. Eur J Appl Physiol. 2000 Mar;81(5):436-42. doi: 10.1007/s004210050065. PMID: 10751106.

'Staying Healthy-Exercising to Relax' by Harvard Health Publishing, July 7, 2020.

Rahman MS, Zhao X, Liu JJ, Torres EQ, Tibert B, Kumar P, Kaldo V, Lindefors N, Forsell Y, Lavebratt C.

Exercise Reduces Salivary Morning CortisolLevels in Patients with Depression. Mol Neuropsychiatry. 2019

REFERENCE MATERIAL – BOOKS AND TEXTS

When the Body Says No, The Cost of Hidden Stress by Gabor Mate

The Power of Now by Eckhart Tolle

Vertical Growth by Michael Bunting and Carl Lemieux

The New Rulebook by Chris Cheers

Manifest by Roxie Nafousi

Reasons Not To Worry-How to be Stoic in Modern Times by Brigid Delaney

Meditations by Marcus Aurelius

Attachment and Loss by John Bowlby

The Adrenal Reset Diet by Dr. Alan Christianson

www.ingramcontent.com/pod-product-compliance
Lightning Source LLC
Chambersburg PA
CBHW070119030426
42335CB00016B/2200